BDJ Clinician's Guides

More information about this series at http://www.springer.com/series/15753

Padhraig Fleming • Jadbinder Seehra

Fixed Orthodontic Appliances

A Practical Guide

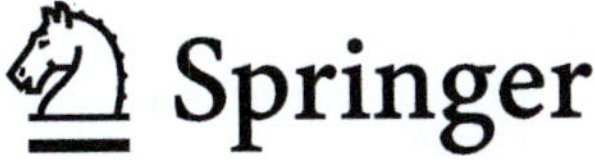

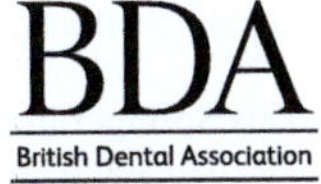

Padhraig Fleming
Orthodontics Department
Queen Mary University of London
London
UK

Jadbinder Seehra
Department of Orthodontics
King's College London
London
UK

Originally published by BDJ Books, London, 2010

ISSN 2523-3327 ISSN 2523-3335 (electronic)
BDJ Clinician's Guides
ISBN 978-3-030-12167-9 ISBN 978-3-030-12165-5 (eBook)
https://doi.org/10.1007/978-3-030-12165-5

Library of Congress Control Number: 2019935820

This Springer imprint is published by the registered company Springer Nature Switzerland AG
The registered company address is: Gewerbestrasse 11, 6330 Cham, Switzerland

Preface

We are privileged to undertake orthodontics on a daily basis. We feel almost uniquely challenged from academic, practical and aesthetic perspectives with an abundance of variables feeding into clinical decision-making. The present text merely scratches the surface of orthodontic care being intended as a practical guide for those starting clinical orthodontics—postgraduates, non-specialist dental providers and orthodontic therapists. As orthodontic educators, we are acutely aware of the challenge of transmitting technical clinical information in an effective and digestible way. We hope that this textbook remedies this problem to an extent and can serve as an essential, basic practical guide during the formative years of clinical orthodontic practice.

Orthodontics is an evolving and progressive specialty. Undeniably, non-specialist provision of care is on the increase; this can of itself be a positive improving access and patient choice. However, a number of proprietary appliance systems have been marketed promising uniquely simple, practical solutions and optimal clinical outcomes with minimal effort or scientific underpinning. Unfortunately, despite the best efforts of orthodontic innovators and the dawn of full appliance customisation, we firmly believe that the clinician rather than his or her tools will continue to be the key determinant of our treatment outcomes. There is, therefore, no substitute either for solid academic grounding or practical understanding and skills. Moreover, the skills and knowledge presented in this textbook are transferable and fundamental to the successful use of an array of fixed appliance systems. Notwithstanding this, we do not consider this textbook to be a stand-alone solution and would recommend deeper learning from allied theoretical and evidence-based books and appropriate in-depth clinical training.

We recognise that clinical manipulation of appliances varies between practitioners and a range of approaches can be applied with unmitigated success. However, we are confident that the techniques that we present have proven successful and predictable over a sustained period. We do hope that you agree and that our clinical approach influences and improves your fixed appliance-based orthodontics.

We would like to express our deepest gratitude to a number of people who have influenced our personal and professional lives. Many of these have engendered a thirst for academic and clinical excellence—others have unwaveringly supported us in this journey. Padhraig would like to pay particular thanks to his wife Caroline and children Ollie, Sophie and Florence Fleming and to his parents (Anne and Johnny).

Jadbinder would also like to acknowledge his father, Pyara Singh Seehra, and his late mother, Mohinder Kaur Seehra. We would both like to thank the numerous friends and colleagues who assisted us with the images presented throughout. We are deeply grateful to Mr. Nick Henchy (American Orthodontics) for providing the stainless steel and aesthetic brackets, archwires and models photographed in the practical sections.

Above all, we hope that you enjoy the book, that it provokes you to think about and improve your practical handling of fixed orthodontic appliances, that it stimulates further and deeper theoretical learning and enquiry and perhaps that it assists in making you a better orthodontic clinician.

London, UK

Padhraig Fleming
Jadbinder Seehra

Contents

Appliance Selection

1

The pre-adjusted edgewise or StraightWire appliance was introduced by Andrews in the 1970s, largely based on occlusal cornerstones derived from analysis of untreated ideals (Andrews 1972). Specifically, Andrews isolated 6 keys to the ideal occlusion based on analysis of 120 non-orthodontic normal occlusions, namely:

- Class I molar relationship
- Correct crown angulation
- Correct crown inclination
- Flat or gentle occlusal curve
- Absence of spacing
- Absence of rotations

The pre-adjusted edgewise brackets were programmed to impart specific prescriptions of tip (second order), torque (third order), in-out and rotational (first order) control on each tooth and reduced the need for wire bending to control tooth position. Numerous variations on Andrew's original prescription have been introduced over the past 30 years (Roth 1987; McLaughlin et al. 2001). Moreover, clinical decisions exist in relation to a range of factors including slot size, mode of ligation and degree of customisation.

In addition, weaknesses in relation to bracket and wire design, manufacturing and metallurgy mean that faithful delivery of prescription is not yet a reality. There is, for example, an acceptance that a 0.019 × 0.025-in. stainless steel wire has approx. 8 degrees of geometric play in a 0.022 × 0.028-in. slot (Gioka and Eliades 2004). Further 'play' arises due to lack of stiffness of wires and brackets, oversized slots, undersized wires and incomplete ligation effectively increasing play by a further 40%. Notwithstanding this, angulation prescription (Table 1.1) tends to be imparted in earlier round wires, while third order (torque; Table 1.2) correction is delivered with rectangular wires.

P. Fleming, J. Seehra, *Fixed Orthodontic Appliances*, BDJ Clinician's Guides,
https://doi.org/10.1007/978-3-030-12165-5_1

Table 1.1 Angulation prescription (in degrees) with popular pre-adjusted edgewise prescriptions. Positive values indicate mesial crown tip

Tooth		1	2	3	4	5	6	7
Maxillary	MBT	4	8	8	0	0	0	0
	Roth	5	9	13	0	0	0	0
	Andrews	5	9	11	2	2	5	5
Mandibular	Andrews	2	2	5	2	2	2	2
	Roth	2	2	7	−1	−1	−1	−1
	MBT	4	8	8	0	0	0	0

Table 1.2 Inclination/torque prescription (in degrees) with popular pre-adjusted edgewise prescriptions. Positive values indicate palatal root torque

Tooth		1	2	3	4	5	6	7
Maxillary	MBT	17	10	0	−7	−7	−14	−14
	Roth	12	8	−2	−7	−7	−14	−14
	Andrews	7	3	−7	−7	−7	−9	−9
Mandibular	Andrews	−1	−1	−11	−17	−22	−30	−30
	Roth	−1	−1	−11	−17	−22	−30	−30
	MBT	−6	−6	−6	−12	−17	−20	−10

1.1 Slot Size: 0.018- or 0.022- In.

Both 0.018-in. and 0.022-in. bracket variants are in common usage. The 0.022-in. system is particularly popular in the UK, although adoption is also increasing in the USA in recent decades with just 40% reporting use of 0.018-in. slots in 2002 (Keim et al. 2002) and self-ligating designs gravitating towards use of the 0.022-in. slot. The 0.022-in. slot allows the potential advantage of stiffer working archwires (0.019 × 0.025″) than with the 0.018-in. system (0.016 × 0.022″). This may facilitate more efficient arch levelling and consequently overbite reduction, although the latter may come at the expense of higher force levels and, therefore, elevated risk of root resorption. Clinical research, however, has shown relatively little impact of bracket dimensions either on treatment duration, quality of result or potential side effects of treatment (Yassir et al. 2018; El-Angbawi et al. 2018).

1.2 Metal or Ceramic Brackets?

Ceramic brackets have been popularised over the past three decades having been introduced in the 1980s offering enhanced aesthetics relative to stainless steel and a potential solution to the problems of other aesthetic variants including plastic brackets (Figs. 1.1–1.3). Early problems in relation to bonding to

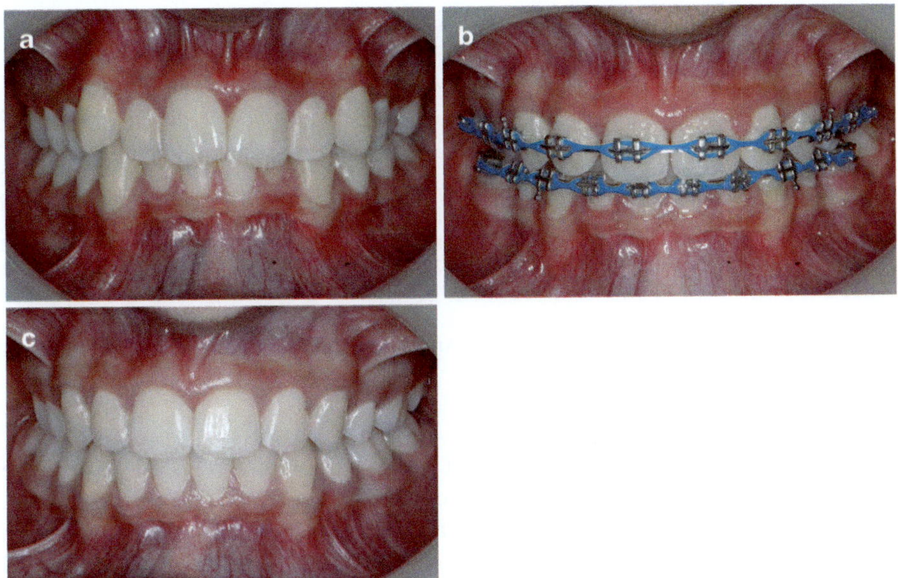

Fig. 1.1 (**a–c**) Stainless steel brackets represent the standard fixed appliance particularly in adolescents with good levels of stiffness, high machinability, good bond strengths and low resistance to sliding

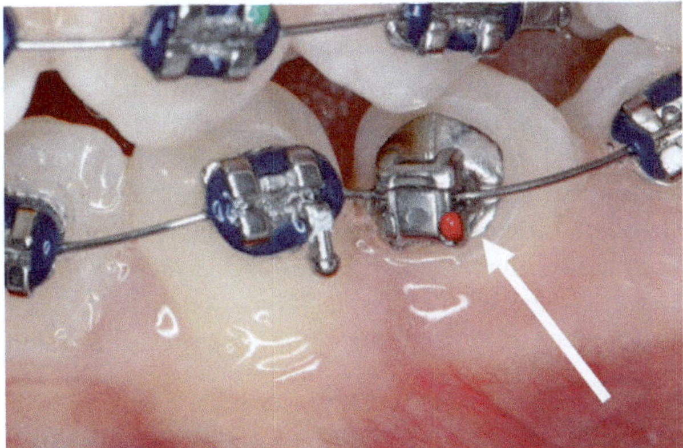

Fig. 1.2 Local use of Damon Q™ self-ligating bracket (arrow) with wire held in place using clip mechanism. There is no evidence that blanket use of self-ligation improves treatment efficiency; however, in areas of significant wire deflection, robust engagement is important and can be problematic with elastomeric materials which tend to fatigue and undergo stress relaxation during intra-oral cycling

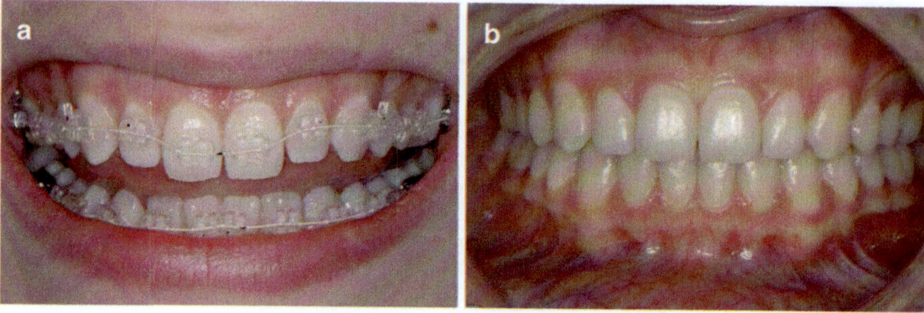

Fig. 1.3 (**a**, **b**) Monocrystalline (Radiance™, American Orthodontics) brackets with high levels of translucency and excellent aesthetics

alumina, an inert material, complicated chemical bonding. This was overcome with use of a silane coupling agent but culminated in stress at the enamel-resin interface and elevated risk of enamel fracture. Consequently, these have been superseded with mechanically retained brackets which have similar bond strengths to metal brackets without risking enamel fracture at debond (Russell 2005).

Ceramic brackets are relatively brittle with lower fracture toughness than stainless steel brackets. Material impurities further reduce this, making the manufacturing process influential. However, ceramic brackets remain more prone to fracture due to occlusal forces and during engagement of large dimension, stiff, rectangular wires.

Ceramic variants (particularly polycrystalline) also have a greater coefficient of friction than stainless steel brackets (Arash et al. 2015). The use of metal inserts may reduce friction compared to conventional ceramic, but not to a level comparable to stainless steel brackets (Cacciafesta et al. 2003). As such, lower fracture toughness and increased friction may affect clinical efficacy; however, laboratory-based studies are not truly representative of the oral environment, and clinical research has identified little meaningful difference in treatment efficiency between these. Ceramic is harder than enamel; therefore, an increased risk of tooth wear exists if used in the lower arch (Russell 2005). As such, disengagement of the occlusion may be necessary to reduce the risk of accelerated wear during treatment.

1.3 Conventional or Self-Ligating Brackets?

Traditionally, steel or elastomeric ligatures have been used to secure the arch wire in the bracket slot, although neither system is ideal. According to Harradine (2003) the ideal bracket ligation system should:

- Be secure and robust.
- Allow the arch wire to be fully engaged in the bracket.
- Have low friction between bracket and arch wire.
- Be quick and easy to use.
- Allow high friction when desired.
- Permit easy attachment of elastic chain.
- Assist good oral hygiene.
- Be comfortable.

Conventional brackets, however, have limitations with respect to ergonomics, efficiency, plastic deformation, discoloration, plaque accumulation and friction. Self-ligating brackets were therefore developed in an attempt to address these shortcomings (Fig. 1.2).

1.4 Choice of Appliance Prescription

Andrews soon recognised that his prescriptions were not universal and soon developed an array of prescriptions based on extraction usage and malocclusion type. Soon, however, the inventory became complicated and was rationed down to a single prescription. Since then, a range of prescriptions have been developed with various increments of torque and angulation values (Roth 1987). Of these, Roth prescription and MBT have become particularly popular in the USA and UK, respectively. Both incorporate more torque in the upper anterior region, likely related to the inefficiency of the fixed system in respect of torque delivery. Roth also incorporated more mesial crown tip in the maxillary canines in order to promote mesial crown positioning and canine guidance; this led to a commensurate increase in anchorage requirements in Class II cases, however. MBT also incorporates more labial root torque (6°) in the lower incisor attachments relative to Andrews or Roth (1°) designed to resist the use of Class II traction in Class II cases and potentially facilitate retraction of lower anteriors in Class III cases. The degree of buccal root torque in the upper buccal segment has also been increased, progressive uprighting torque added to the lower molars and increased torque options provided for the maxillary canines (McLaughlin and Bennett 2015).

1.5 Customised or Non-customised Brackets

Andrews' StraightWire system was the first to introduce a degree of customisation within the brackets with correction in terms of in-out and rotational control (first order) with control of bracket thickness and base morphology. Angulation (second order) and torque (third order) were imparted by virtue of orientation of the bracket slot. These prescriptions have permitted adequate levels of control and precision; however, full customisation of labial and lingual systems has come into vogue in recent years. The latter involves indirect fabrication and placement of appliances with bespoke customisation of individual teeth. Workflow tends to change accordingly with non-clinical time potentially increasing and chairside time reducing. These bespoke appliances also tend to be costlier to fabricate. Significant benefit has not been demonstrated in clinical research with no significant difference in terms of treatment duration or quality of outcome (Penning et al. 2017), although customisation of lingual appliances may offer more fundamental benefit in view of the inter-individual variation in lingual tooth surface morphology.

Box 1.1 Development of Fixed Appliance Systems

Edward Angle is credited with developing the early fixed appliance systems. He is regarded as 'The father of orthodontics' developing an array of dental devices with 14 patents to his name ranging from orthodontic appliances to farm implements (Peck 2009). Angle's most enduring and influential discovery was the Standard Edgewise system which he developed in 1928 (Angle 1928). He described this as 'the latest and the best' of a series of appliances that he designed. It received its name as the archwire which was introduced horizontally (on its edge) for the first time—previous systems had involved vertical insertion of the wire. Angle's Edgewise system was machined from gold predating the adoption of stainless steel.

Standard edgewise lacked prescription in the attachment themselves; as such, artistic wire bending was obligatory in order to compensate for differences in tooth thicknesses, vertical slot positioning, angulation and torque. Adjustment was therefore laborious; moreover, the appliance was predicated on Angle's conviction that malocclusion was environmental in origin and uniformly amenable to non-extraction treatment. One of Angle's disciples, Raymond Begg, however, based on analysis of Aboriginal diet and occlusal characteristics came to believe that extraction-based treatment was required to compensate for lack of attrition and diminution of jaw size associated with modern diets (Begg 1954). He subsequently developed the eponymous Begg appliance which became popular in the UK, Australasia and parts of the USA.

It was not until Andrews' refinement of Angle's original designs that the Edgewise system became universally popular. It should be noted, however, that Angle himself was aware of the possibility of altering bracket orientation rather than wire morphology utilising wires 'freest from bends' to simplify and improve the precision of fixed appliances. However, Angle died in 1930; he may have realised this ambition himself had he survived longer.

Box 1.2 Limitations of StraightWire Appliance

Early adopters of the StraightWire appliance (SWA) recognised inherent limitations related to specific prescriptions. In particular, mesial angulation built into the appliance may have an effect on antero-posterior and vertical tooth positioning. Expression of mesial tip in the canine brackets tends to exert an extrusive effect on the anterior teeth potentially leading to an increased overbite. This can be controlled with mechanics either early or later in treatment. Furthermore, mesial tip in the posterior segments, but particularly the canines, risks loss of posterior anchorage leading to mesial movement of the buccal segments. Preludes to the StraightWire appliance had included the Begg (and later Tip-Edge™) system which involved early use of inter-arch elastics on round wires to produce free distal tipping of maxillary canines in Class II cases. The anchorage issues associated with the SWA, therefore, deterred wider adoption in its earlier years. Obviously, the pre-adjusted system also lacks full customisation; however, an understanding of bracket prescriptions allows for some flexibility and use of local bracket variation to address specific issues (Thickett et al. 2007). A whole range of variations can be used (Table 1.3) with the effect of angulation and inclination changes being quite potent (Fig. 1.4a–c).

Table 1.3 More common local bracket variations with associated rationale and indications

Variation	Rationale	Indication
Inversion maxillary lateral incisor	Additional labial root torque	Palatal lateral incisor
Reverse lower canine	Additional distal crown tip	Control lower arch length, e.g. in Class III camouflage
Inversion of maxillary canine bracket	Additional palatal root torque (pending on prescription)	Buccally placed maxillary canine
Maxillary premolar bracket on maxillary canine (or intentional mesial angulation of canine bracket)	Limit mesial crown tipping and associated anchorage demand to move root distally	Class II cases where anchorage at a premium in maxillary arch
Inversion of MBT™ mandibular incisor bracket™	Additional lingual root torque	Thin gingival biotype with lower labial recession where lingual root positioning may be beneficial
Inversion of mandibular premolar brackets	Additional lingual root torque	Scissors bite where mandibular arch expansion may improve transverse co-ordination
Inversion of maxillary premolar brackets	Additional palatal root torque	Posterior crossbite where maxillary arch expansion may improve transverse co-ordination

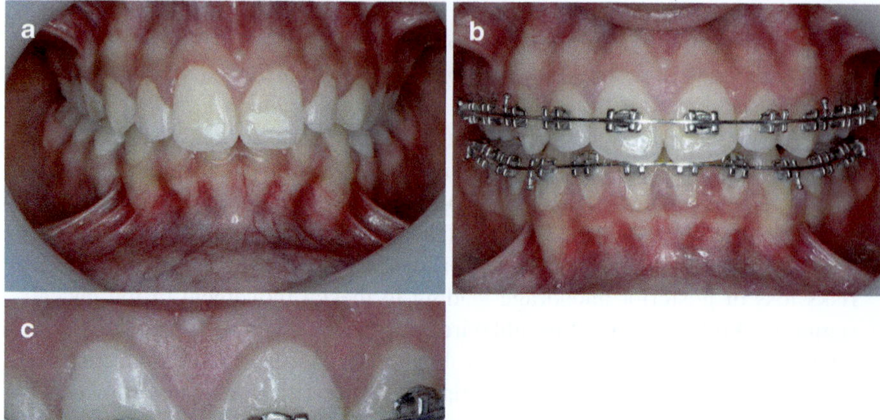

Fig. 1.4 (**a**–**c**) A bracket positioning error with inadvertent reversal of the maxillary central incisor Roth brackets. The intended 5 degrees of mesial crown tip has been converted into distal tip leading to a second-order issue. This can be rectified either with wire bending or bracket repositioning

Box 1.3 Friction in Fixed Appliance Systems

Friction is defined as the resistance to motion when an object moves tangentially against another. Low friction may be desirable to expedite efficient alignment and space closure while keeping anchorage requirements low. Occasionally high friction is preferable limiting unwanted tooth movement and facilitating torque delivery (Harradine 2003; Pandis et al. 2006). Research on frictional resistance to orthodontic tooth movement in vivo is complex; our knowledge is almost entirely based on laboratory-based investigations using simulated oral environments involving salivary substitutes and intermittent jiggling forces similar to masticatory forces.

It is difficult to determine the correlation between artificial laboratory-based set-ups and the in vivo situation. However, the importance of friction within orthodontic appliances in vivo is debated (Braun et al. 1999; Burrow 2009). Indeed, although a reduced-friction appliance may be expected to produce more rapid, efficient alignment, rotational correction and space closure, there is no published clinical evidence to confirm this (Hain et al. 2003).

Masticatory activity may diminish the impact of frictional resistance within an orthodontic appliance system in vivo with an estimated reduction of 80% in a 0.019 × 0.025-in. stainless steel wire (O'Reilly et al. 1999). The authors concluded that the importance of friction in orthodontic appliances might be overstated.

Box 1.4 Lingual or Labial Appliances

Labial fixed appliance systems form the mainstay of fixed appliance treatment as these are relatively simple to manufacture, place and manipulate. They do, however, have the clear disadvantage of being visible with resultant aesthetic impairment, allied to potential enamel demineralisation on more visible tooth surfaces. Lingual orthodontics is complicated by issues relating to access but also, more fundamentally, morphological variation of the lingual surfaces of teeth. As such, customisation of bracket bases and adhesive has been undertaken with indirect bonding of brackets to facilitate appliance placement (Fig. 1.5a–c). Evidence concerning the relative effectiveness of each is fairly equivocal and should be tempered by the knowledge that lingual users typically graduate to using these systems following previous experience with labial systems. Overall treatment time is likely to be slightly longer with lingual systems, although evidence in this respect is not compelling. In terms of patient experiences, discomfort tends to be more severe and slightly more protracted (up to 14 days) with lingual appliances being focussed on the tongue rather than labial and buccal mucosa (Wu et al. 2009), and speech impairment for up to 14 days is also typical.

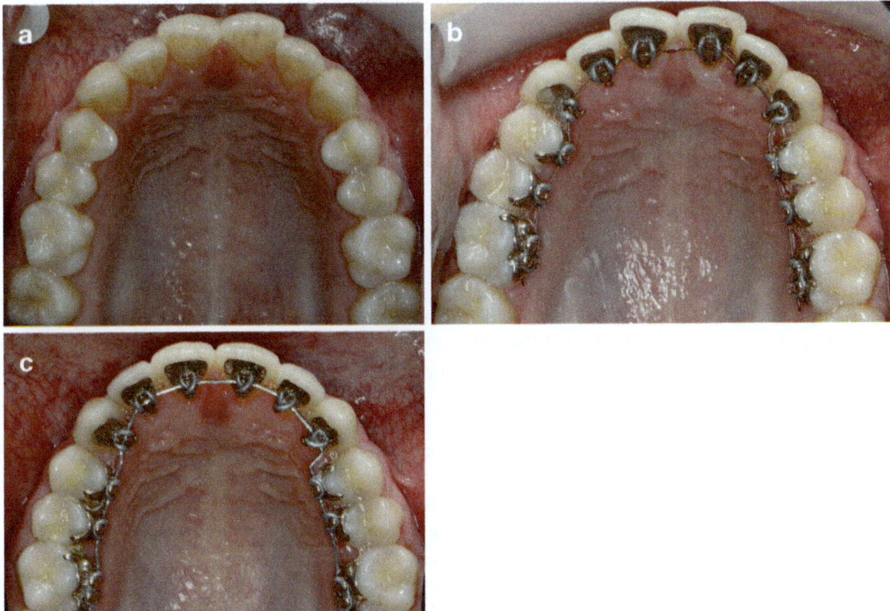

Fig. 1.5 (**a–c**) Customised lingual orthodontic appliances with bespoke bracket base design and morphology permitting improved predictability in terms of bonding and tooth movement. Customisation can be applied to the bracket (Incognito™) or adhesive base (WIN™) simplifying wire formation and reducing the onus on wire bending at chairside

References

Andrews LF. The six keys to normal occlusion. Am J Orthod. 1972;62(3):296–309.

Angle EH. The latest and best in orthodontic mechanism. Dental Cosmos. 1928;70:1143–58.

Arash V, Rabiee M, Rakhshan V, Khorasani S, Sobouti F. In vitro evaluation of frictional forces of two ceramic orthodontic brackets versus a stainless steel bracket in combination with two types of archwires. J Orthod Sci. 2015;4(2):42–6.

Begg PR. Stone Age man's dentition: with reference to anatomically correct occlusion, the etiology of malocclusion, and a technique for its treatment. Am J Orthod. 1954;40(4):298–312.

Braun S, Bluestein M, Moore BK, Benson G. Friction in perspective. Am J Orthod Dentofac Orthop. 1999;115(6):619–27.

Burrow SJ. Friction and resistance to sliding in orthodontics: a critical review. Am J Orthod Dentofac Orthop. 2009;135(4):442–7.

Cacciafesta V, Sfondrini MF, Ricciardi A, Scribante A, Klersy C, Auricchio F. Evaluation of friction of stainless steel and esthetic self-ligating brackets in various bracket-archwire combinations. Am J Orthod Dentofac Orthop. 2003;124(4):395–402.

El-Angbawi AM, Yassir YA, McIntyre GT, Revie GF, Bearn DR. A randomized clinical trial of the effectiveness of 0.018-inch and 0.022-inch slot orthodontic bracket systems: part 3—biological side-effects of treatment. Eur J Orthod. 2018. https://doi.org/10.1093/ejo/cjy039.

Gioka C, Eliades T. Materials-induced variation in the torque expression of preadjusted appliances. Am J Orthod Dentofac Orthop. 2004;125(3):323–8.

Hain M, Dhopatkar A, Rock P. The effect of ligation method on friction in sliding mechanics. Am J Orthod Dentofac Orthop. 2003;123(4):416–22.

Harradine NW. Self-ligating brackets: where are we now? J Orthod. 2003;30(3):262–73.

Keim RG, Gottlieb EL, Nelson AH. 2002 JCO study of orthodontic diagnosis and treatment procedures. Part 2. Breakdowns of selected variables. J Clin Orthod. 2002;36(11):627–36.

McLaughlin RP, Bennett JC. Evolution of treatment mechanics and contemporary appliance design in orthodontics: a 40-year perspective. Am J Orthod Dentofac Orthop. 2015;147(6):654–62.

McLaughlin RP, Bennett JC, Trevisi HJ. Systemized orthodontic treatment mechanics. St. Louis: Elsevier Health Sciences; 2001.

O'Reilly D, Dowling PA, Lagerstrom L, Swartz ML. An ex vivo investigation into the effect of bracket displacement on the resistance to sliding. J Orthod. 1999;26(3):219–27.

Pandis N, et al. Maxillary incisor torque with conventional and self-ligating brackets: a prospective clinical trial. Orthod Craniofac Res. 2006;9(4):193–8.

Peck S. A biographical portrait of Edward Hartley Angle, the first specialist in orthodontics, part 1. Angle Orthod. 2009;79(6):1021–7.

Penning EW, Peerlings RH, Govers JD, Rischen RJ, Zinad K, Bronkhorst EM, Breuning KH, Kuijpers-Jagtman AM. Orthodontics with customized versus noncustomized appliances: a randomized controlled clinical trial. J Dent Res. 2017;96(13):1498–504.

Roth RH. The straight-wire appliance 17 years later. J Clin Orthod. 1987;21(9):632–42.

Russell JS. Current products and practice: aesthetic orthodontic brackets. J Orthod. 2005;32(2):146–63.

Thickett E, Taylor NG, Hodge T. Choosing a pre-adjusted orthodontic appliance prescription for anterior teeth. J Orthod. 2007;34(2):95–100.

Wu AK, McGrath C, Wong RW, Wiechmann D, Rabie ABM. A comparison of pain experienced by patients treated with labial and lingual orthodontic appliances. Eur J Orthod. 2009;32(4):403–7.

Yassir YA, El-Angbawi AM, McIntyre GT, Revie GF, Bearn DR. A randomized clinical trial of the effectiveness of 0.018-inch and 0.022-inch slot orthodontic bracket systems: part 2—quality of treatment. Eur J Orthod. 2018. https://doi.org/10.1093/ejo/cjy038.

2 Orthodontic Instruments

Orthodontic instruments are specifically designed to facilitate orthodontic treatment. Like most instruments used in dental specialties, they are usually made from stainless steel, are unique and have a specific design and purpose. Although not exhaustive, the following is a description of commonly used orthodontic instruments and equipment.

Stainless steel mouth mirror (Fig. 2.1a, b)

- Access for both direct and indirect vision
- Checking bracket position and placement (Fig. 2.1c, d)
- Soft tissue retraction during examination, placement and removal of fixed appliance attachments (Fig. 2.1e)

Short dental probe (Fig. 2.2a, b)

- Examination of tooth surfaces and restorations
- Positioning of orthodontic attachments
- Removal of composite flash
- Removal of elastomeric ties from bracket tie-wings with the probe normally pointed in an occlusal direction (Fig. 2.2c, d)

College tweezers (Fig. 2.3a, b)

- Retrieval of small fragments from within the oral cavity
- May facilitate aseptic transfer of small instruments and placement of bonded retainers

P. Fleming, J. Seehra, *Fixed Orthodontic Appliances*, BDJ Clinician's Guides,
https://doi.org/10.1007/978-3-030-12165-5_2

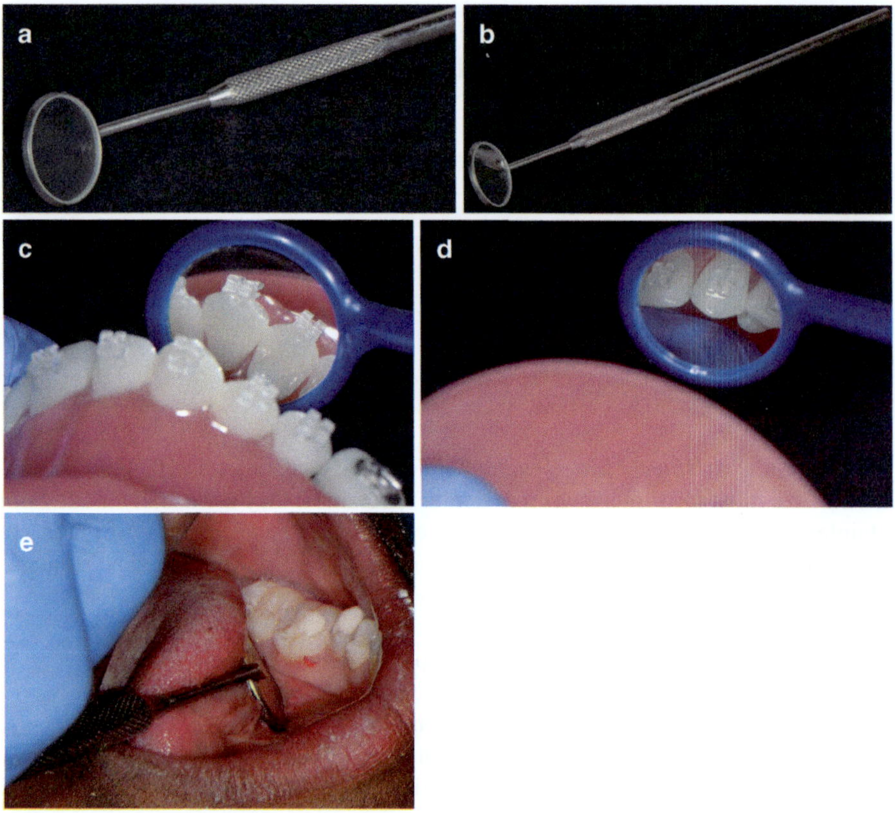

Fig. 2.1 (**a**–**e**) Stainless steel mouth mirror

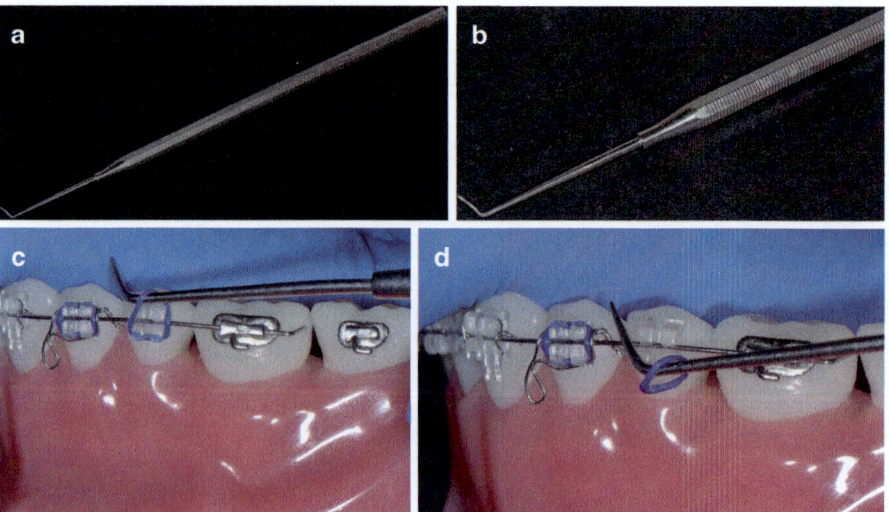

Fig. 2.2 (**a**–**d**) Short dental probe

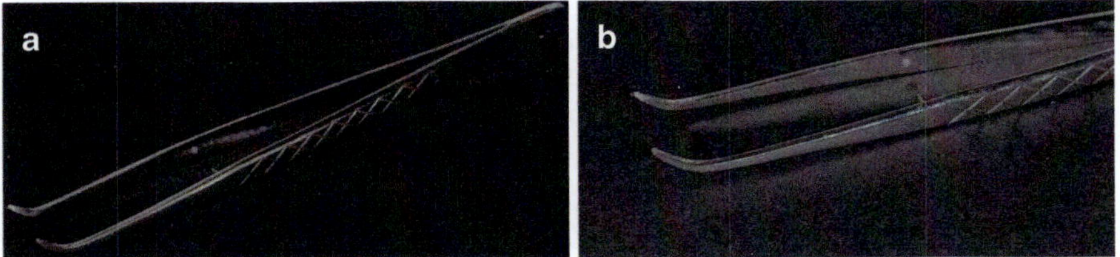

Fig. 2.3 (**a**, **b**) College tweezers

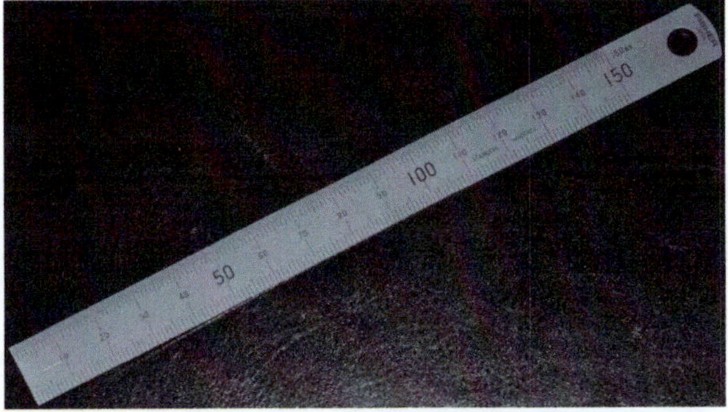

Fig. 2.4 Ruler

Ruler (Fig. 2.4)

- Used in the assessment of overjet, level of crowding (ideally with a clear ruler) and treatment progress, particularly in relation to transverse arch dimensional changes

Ligature director (Fig. 2.5a–c)

- Tucking the ends of wire auxiliaries (lacebacks, short or long ligatures and Kobayashi ligatures) away from the soft tissues and beneath the archwire
- Engagement of Nickel-Titanium archwires into the bracket slot of rotated or displaced teeth

Weingart pliers (Fig. 2.6a, b)

- Directing larger dimension round and rectangular archwires through molar bands and tubes
- Squeezing crimpable stops onto archwires

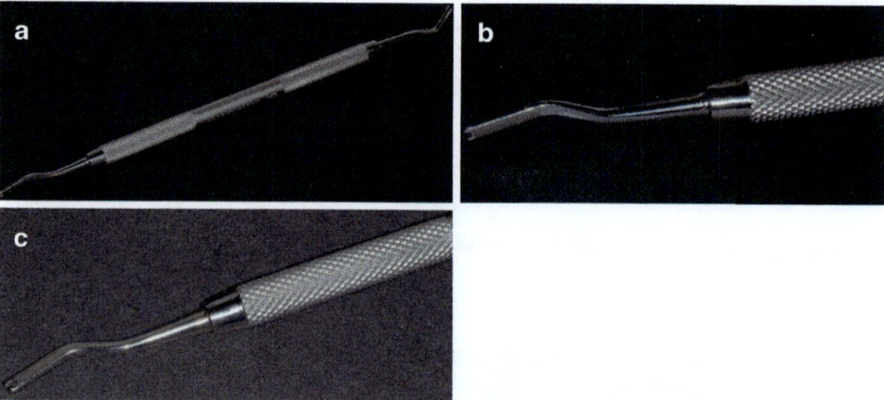

Fig. 2.5 (**a**–**c**) Ligature director

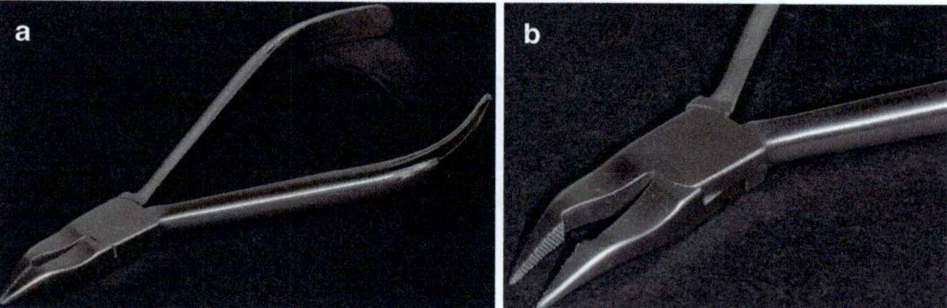

Fig. 2.6 (**a**, **b**) Weingart pliers

Light wire pliers (Fig. 2.7a, b)

- Directing larger dimension round and rectangular archwires through distal molar attachments
- Wire bending including closing loops, first- and second-order finishing bends in round (0.016-, 0.018- and 0.020-in.) and rectangular stainless steel archwires or Beta- Titanium archwires (0.017 × 25- , 0.018 × 25- and 0.019 × 25-in.)

Posterior band remover (Fig. 2.8a, b)

- Removal of molar and premolar bands

Mershon band pusher (Fig. 2.9a, b)

- Seating of molar and premolar bands through the contact points of adjacent teeth
- Burnishing the edges of bands against tooth surface to improve both adaptation and fit

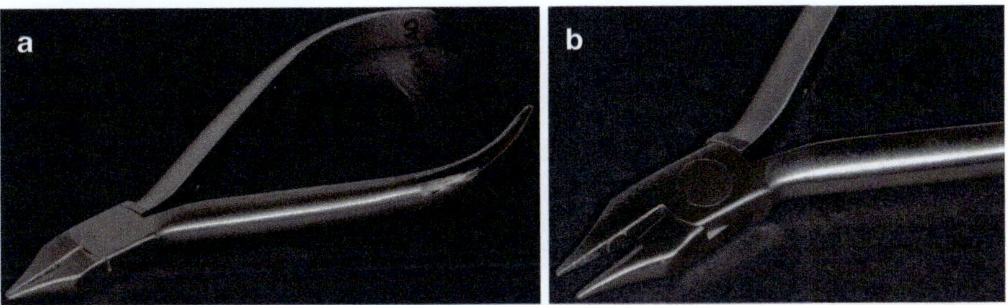

Fig. 2.7 (**a**, **b**) Light wire pliers

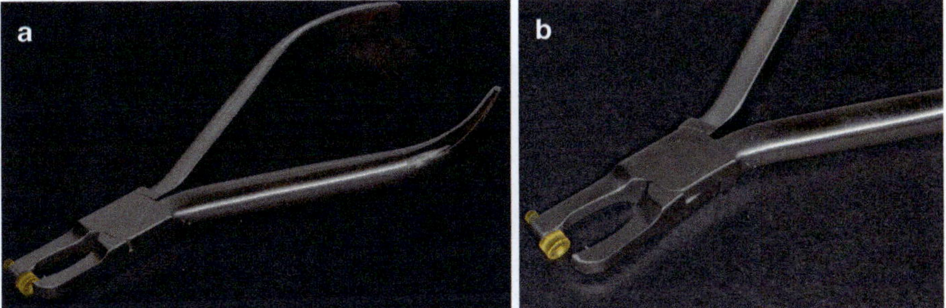

Fig. 2.8 (**a**, **b**) Posterior band remover

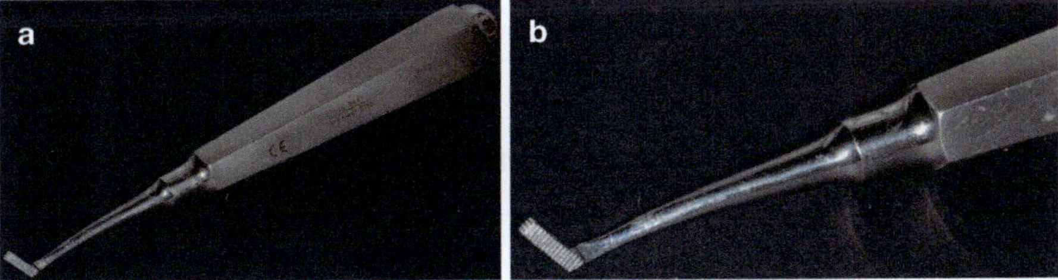

Fig. 2.9 (**a**, **b**) Mershon band pusher

Direct metal bracket debonding pliers (Fig. 2.10a, b)

- Removal of orthodontic brackets and tubes from the surface of the teeth through application of shearing force resulting in failure between the adhesive layer and bracket base

Direct bond bracket tweezers (Fig. 2.11a, b)

- Positioning of orthodontic brackets and attachments directly onto the buccal surfaces of the teeth

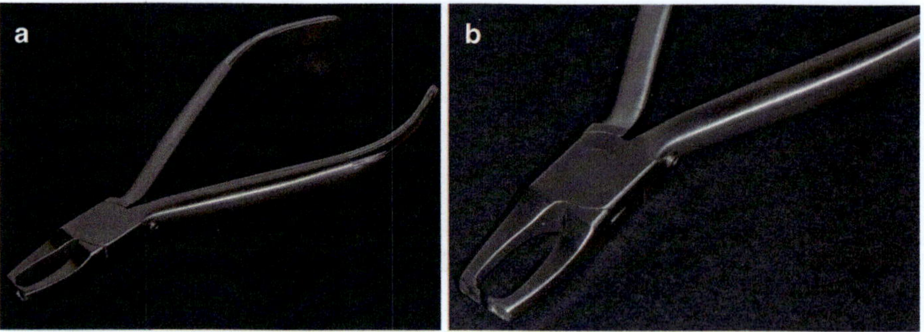

Fig. 2.10 (**a**, **b**) Direct metal bracket debonding pliers

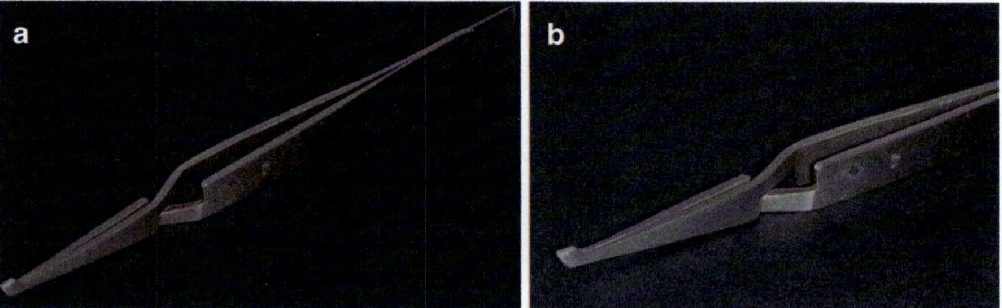

Fig. 2.11 (**a**, **b**) Direct bond bracket tweezers

Buccal tube tweezers (Fig. 2.12a–c)

- Positioning of buccal molar tubes on upper and lower permanent molar teeth

Mosquito forceps (Fig. 2.13)

- Placement of elastomerics around the bracket tie-wings to secure the archwire into the bracket slot
- Placement of separator elastics
- Securing stainless steel short, long and Kobayashi ligatures, although alternatives including Mathieu forceps are commonly used

These are available with either curved or straight serrated beaks with a locking mechanism between the forceps handles. Curved forceps may be more useful in lingual orthodontics, particularly posteriorly.

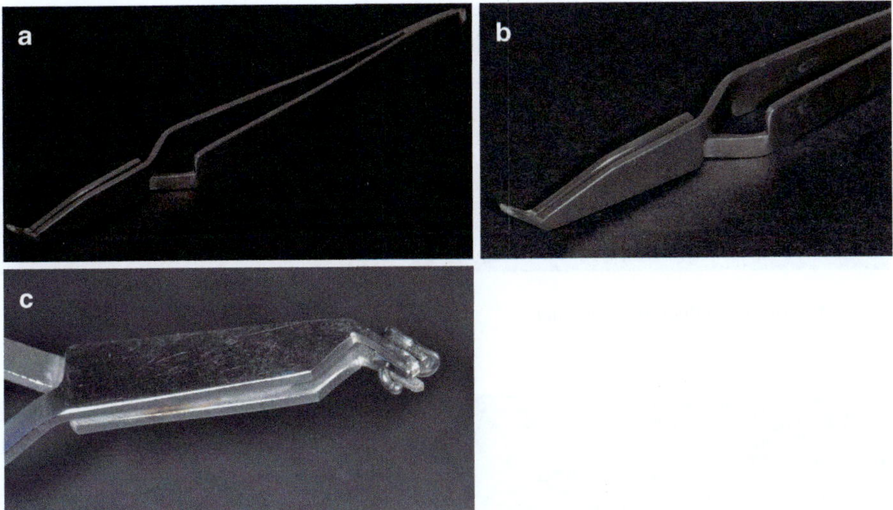

Fig. 2.12 (**a–c**) Buccal tube tweezers

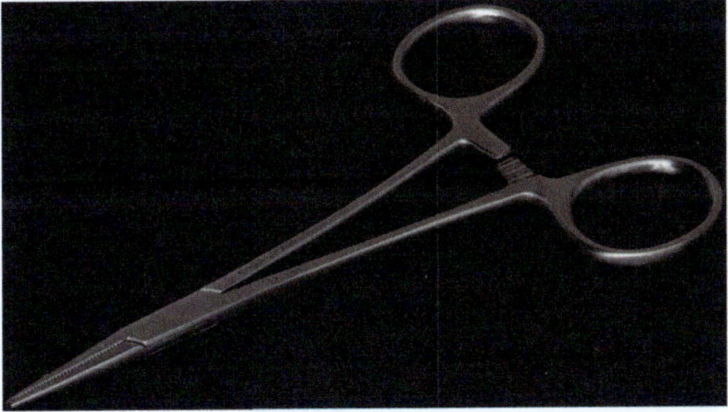

Fig. 2.13 Mosquito forceps

Mathieu forceps/pliers (Fig. 2.14a, b)

- Placement of stainless steel short, long and Kobayashi ligatures around the tie-wings of the brackets

These are similar to mosquito forceps but are commonly available with opposing straight serrated beaks and have a locking mechanism between the forceps handles

Ligature cutter (Fig. 2.15a, b)

- Cutting ends of stainless steel short, long and Kobayashi ligatures following ligation around the bracket tie-wings

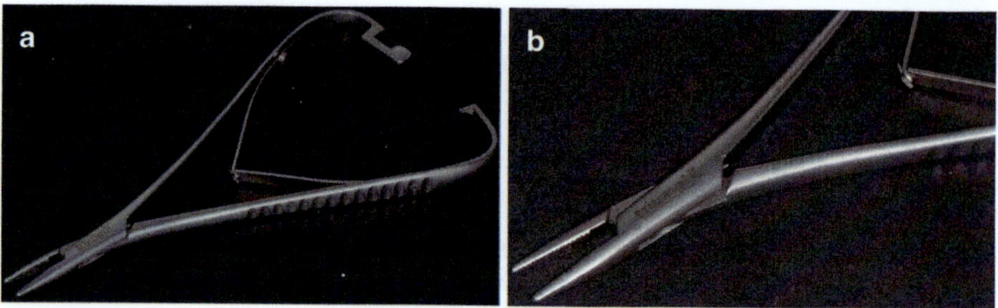

Fig. 2.14 (**a**, **b**) Mathieu forceps/pliers

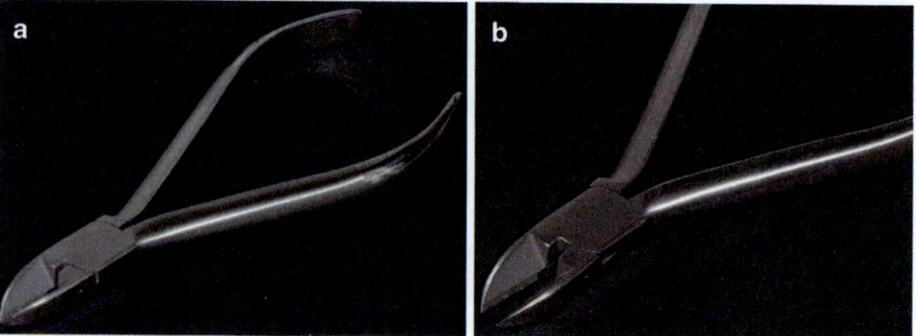

Fig. 2.15 (**a**, **b**) Ligature cutter

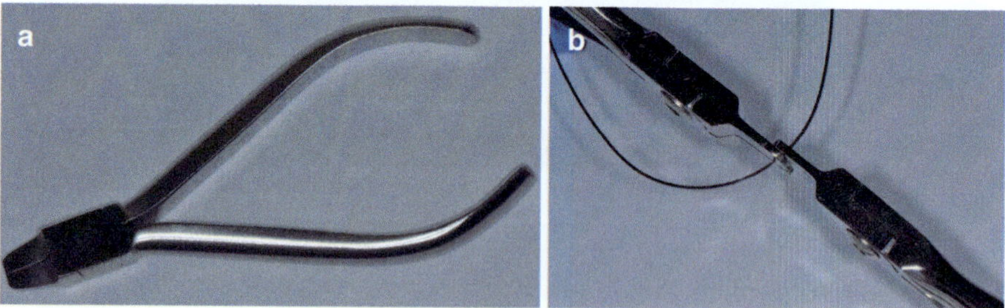

Fig. 2.16 (**a**, **b**) Tweed rectangular arch forming pliers

Tweed rectangular arch forming pliers (Fig. 2.16a)

- Wire bending such as first-, second- and third-order bends in rectangular stainless steel and Beta-Titanium archwires (0.017 × 25-, 0.018 × 25- and 0.019 × 25-in.)
- Two tweed rectangular arch forming pliers may be used to introduce third-order (torque) bends (Fig. 2.16b)

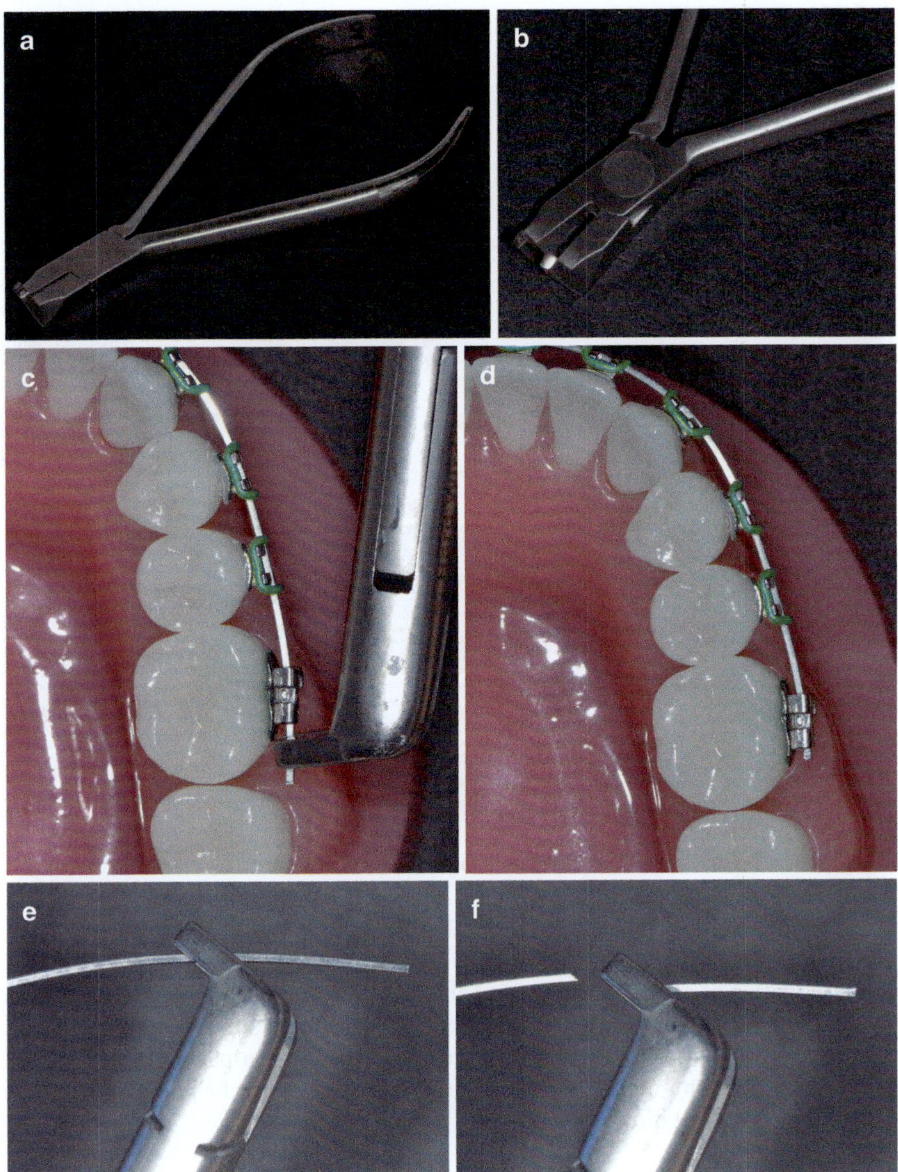

Fig. 2.17 (**a**–**f**) Distal end cutter

Distal end cutter (Fig. 2.17a, b)

- Cutting the distal end of round and rectangular Nickel-Titanium and stainless steel archwires once passed through molar attachments such as molar bands and tubes (Fig. 2.17c, d)

These include a safety feature gripping the distal fragment of the archwire once the wire has been cut to length (Fig. 2.17e, f).

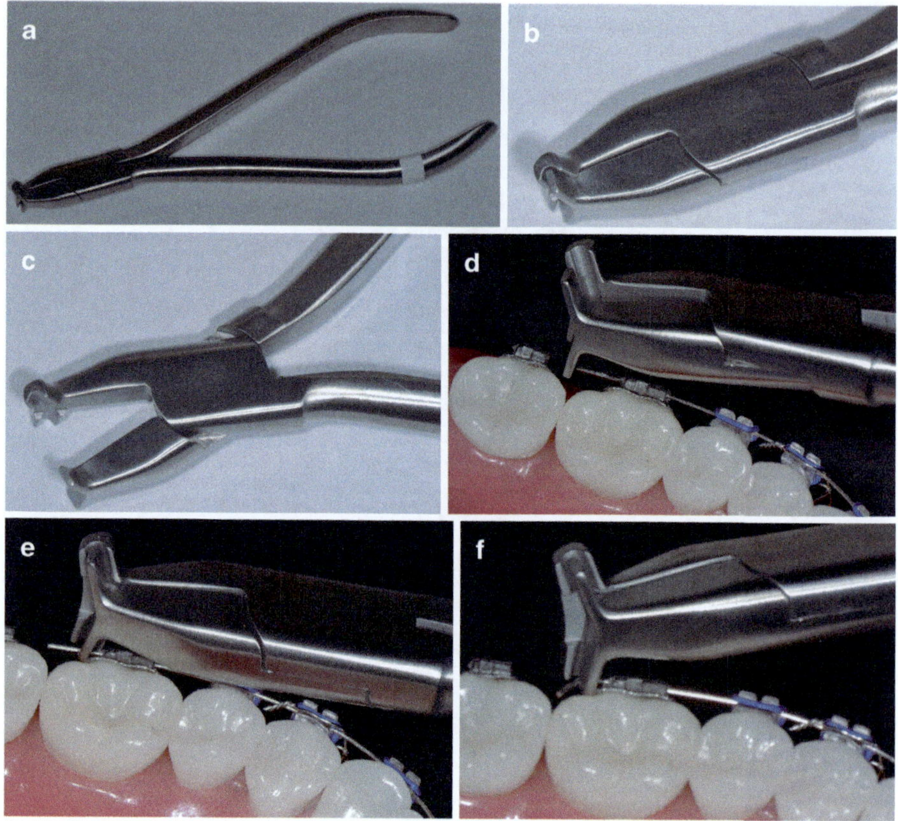

Fig. 2.18 (**a–f**) Hammerhead Nickel-Titanium tie-back (Cinch) pliers

Hammerhead Nickel-Titanium tie-back (Cinch) pliers (Fig. 2.18a–c)

- Introduction of acute bends in round and rectangular Nickel-Titanium archwires. Wires can be bent in a lingual direction away from the soft tissues and towards the contact point between the teeth once they have been passed through distal molar attachments (Fig. 2.18d–f). Alternatively, a bend can be placed moving the wire in a gingival direction.

Chinagraph marker/pencils (Fig. 2.19)

– Marking the location of first-, second- and third-order archwire bends and/or auxiliaries such as crimpable stops or hooks onto the archwire

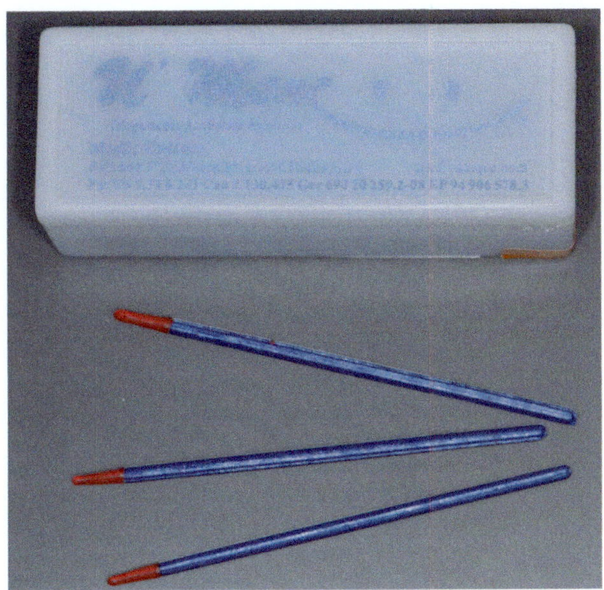

Fig. 2.19 Chinagraph marker/pencils

Bracket Placement and Positioning

3

The introduction of the acid-etch technique within dentistry has influenced modern orthodontic bonding techniques (Buonocore 1955) prompting a move away from multi-banded appliances which characterised pioneering standard edgewise and Begg techniques. Bonding has helped to simplify and expedite appliance placement while improving comfort and hygiene. As such, bonded attachments are typically preferred, although banded molar attachments may be required in conjunction with banded appliances including fixed expansion auxiliaries and transpalatal and lingual arches. However, clinical research has largely failed to show a benefit of molar bonding in terms of demineralisation, patient comfort or failure rates (Nazir et al. 2011).

The optimal bond strength to retain orthodontic attachments to the enamel surfaces has been estimated at 5.9–7.8 MPa and is dependent on bonding techniques (Reynolds and von Fraunhofer 1976). The choice of fixed appliance used in a particular case to deliver the treatment aims and objectives should be decided at the treatment planning stage based on an appreciation of prescriptions (Tables 1.1 and 1.2), treatment objectives, availability of space and anchorage requirements. Correct bracket positioning facilitates efficient treatment and may reduce the duration of the finishing stage of treatment (Chap. 8) and the need for additional wire bending (Chap. 9).

P. Fleming, J. Seehra, *Fixed Orthodontic Appliances*, BDJ Clinician's Guides,
https://doi.org/10.1007/978-3-030-12165-5_3

Box 3.1 Direct Bracket Placement and Common Errors

When positioning orthodontic brackets directly onto the tooth surface, the following factors should be considered: base adaptation, slot angulation and mesio-distal (rotational) and vertical position (Carlson and Johnson 2001). Ensuring that the bracket base is well-contoured against the tooth surface helps to promote an even layer of adhesive. Failure to seat the bracket completely can lead to unwanted rotational effects (Fig. 3.1a, b). Tooth-related factors such as shape, size, morphology, eruption, lingual/palatal position and gingival height should also be considered. Direct bonding is associated with errors in bracket angulation and inclination (Taylor and Cook 1992). Adjunctive measures such as bracket gauges (Fig. 3.2a, b) which use the incisal edge for incisors and the occlusal plane for posterior teeth as a reference point can be used to aid vertical bracket placement (Armstrong et al. 2007).

Brackets should normally be positioned in the centre of the clinical crown (long-axis or LA point) with the tie-wings perpendicular to the long axis of the tooth. Alternative designs do exist with gingival offsetting of premolar brackets, for example, used to mitigate against a tendency to position these in an occlusal position. By convention, the disto-gingival tie-wing is highlighted (either in colour or with a small indentation) to orientate the bracket correctly (Fig. 3.3a, b); both gingival tie-wings can be highlighted in brackets that can be placed interchangeably on left and right sides (including some mandibular incisors and premolars with 0° angulation).

The centre of the clinical crown is considered to be reproducible despite individual tooth variation. However, anomalies in tooth length related to incisal wear and gingival architecture issues may need to be accounted for with attachments being placed at the centre of the ideal anatomic crown in these cases particularly where gingival recontouring or direct bonding is planned. Where incisal edge reduction (disking) is planning to compensate for uneven wear, brackets may intentionally be positioned gingival to the LA point to extrude the tooth prior to reshaping. As a guide, the long axis of the tooth should bisect the middle of the bracket base (Fig. 3.4) with the vertical reference line on the bracket being used to guide the mesio-distal orientation along the long axis.

For the placement of molar tube attachments, the same principles as with molar bands should be adhered to. For maxillary and mandibular first molars, the tube should be bonded adjacent to the buccal groove and mesio-buccal groove, respectively, parallel to the buccal cusps with an even amount of the mesial and distal cusps visible (Fig. 3.5). Optimal bracket placement is critical in avoiding alignment issues towards the end of treatment (see Chaps. 8 and 9). Common specific bracket errors and their resultant effect on tooth position are highlighted in Table 3.1 (McLaughlin et al. 2001).

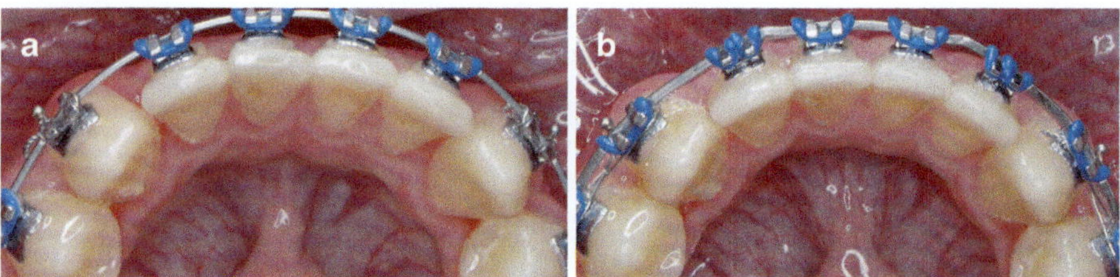

Fig. 3.1 (**a**, **b**) Failure to seat the LR1 and LL1 brackets has resulted in an excessive, uneven layer of adhesive beneath each bracket base. Engagement of a lower rectangular Nickel-Titanium archwire highlights the rotational errors (**a**). A lower rectangular Beta-Titanium archwire with first-order correction bends is ligated to address the position of LR1 and LL1 (**b**)

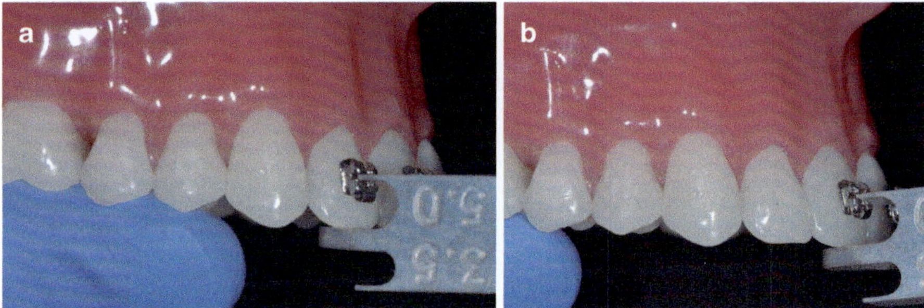

Fig. 3.2 (**a**, **b**) A bracket gauge being used to guide vertical bracket placement using the maxillary central incisor edge as a reference point

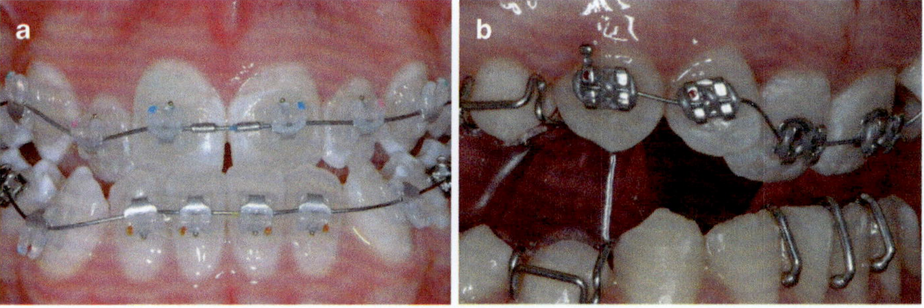

Fig. 3.3 (**a**, **b**) Disto-gingival demarcation on anterior brackets to assist with identification

Fig. 3.4 The vertical reference line on the bracket is used to guide the mesio-distal orientation along the long axis of the clinical crown

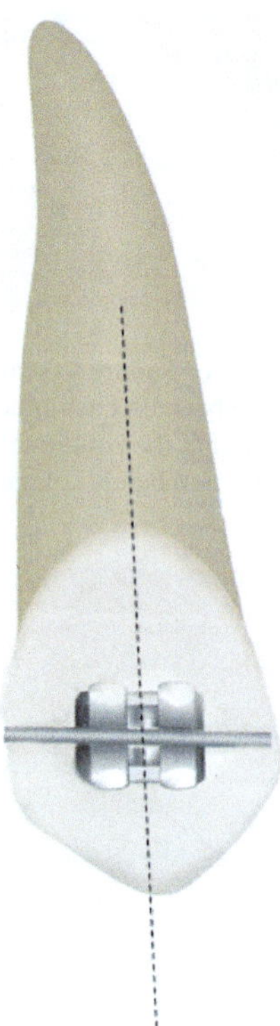

Fig. 3.5 Maxillary first molar tubes should be centred on the buccal groove parallel to the buccal cusps

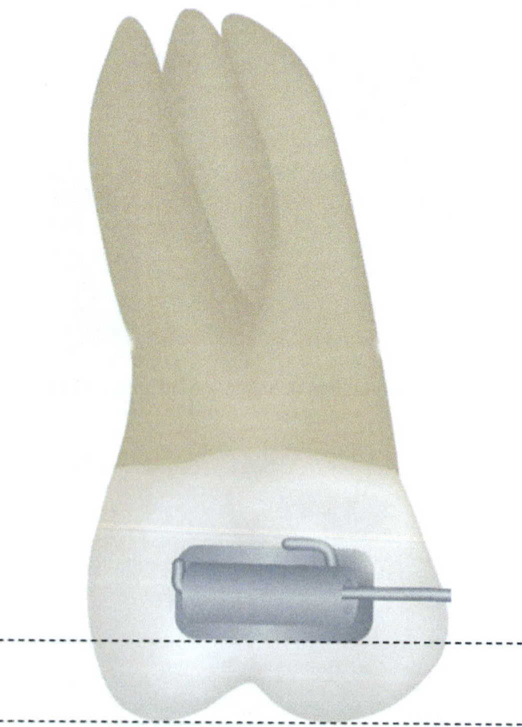

Table 3.1 Common bracket positioning errors and their effect on tooth position

Tooth	Error (s)	Effect
Maxillary central incisors	Bracket not positioned parallel to long axis of the tooth	Angulation and associated rotational discrepancy
Maxillary lateral incisors	Bracket placed too incisally	Intrusion and increased vertical step between incisal edges of adjacent maxillary central incisor and canine
Maxillary canines	Horizontal positioning	Rotational discrepancy
Maxillary premolar	Bracket placed too occlusal	Intrusion of the tooth resulting in marginal ridge discrepancies between adjacent molar and poor buccal occlusion interdigitation
Maxillary first molars	Molar tube/band placed too gingival (particularly over-seating palatally)	Extrusion of the tooth resulting in marginal ridge discrepancies between adjacent premolar, poor buccal occlusion interdigitation and reduction in overbite
Mandibular canines	Horizontal positioning: Usually distal	Rotational discrepancy (mesio-lingual), which may complicate fixed retainer placement unless corrected
Mandibular premolars	Bracket placed too occlusal	Intrusion of the tooth resulting in marginal ridge discrepancies between adjacent molar and poor buccal occlusion interdigitation
Mandibular first molars	Molar tube/band placed too gingival	Extrusion of the tooth resulting in marginal ridge discrepancies between adjacent premolar and poor buccal occlusion interdigitation. Lingual crown inclination can also develop

Box 3.2 Intentional Variation in Bracket Placement

In certain malocclusions, in different stages of treatment or to facilitate particular tooth movements, bracket placement can be varied from the 'ideal' positions. During initial positioning of brackets, the centre of the clinical crown may not be accessible due to the level of crowding, rotations and overlap of the adjacent teeth. In these situations, the bracket can initially be bonded in a non-ideal position (usually mesial or distal to the long axis) before being moved into the correct position following initial alignment (Fig. 3.6a–d).

During the alignment stage, it may be important to maintain the arch length to avoid excess proclination of the lower incisors leading to arch length changes with resultant change in the overbite and overjet. For example, in the lower arch in Class III camouflage, the contralateral lower canine brackets can be bonded to maintain the lower arch length. This changes the prescribed 3° mesial tip (with the MBT system) to distal tip encouraging distal crown tipping relative to the root and control of the antero-posterior position of the lower labial segment (Fig. 3.6e–j). Cinching the archwire flush against the distal aspect of the molar attachment can also help to maintain the arch length; however, the latter does not affect canine angulation.

Where one or both upper lateral incisors are developmentally absent, substituting the upper permanent canines in the upper lateral incisor position can be considered along with space closure (Silveira et al. 2016). In this situation, the upper canine bracket which has labial root torque prescription can be inverted to move the root palatally and optimise gingival aesthetics (Fig. 3.6k–t). It is important that a canine bracket with a meaningful amount of torque (e.g. Andrews or MBT variants) is used to have a demonstrable effect.

Where the maxillary lateral incisors have erupted palatally, often the most challenging and time-consuming treatment objective is labial movement of the roots of these teeth. This is complicated further by the fact the torque prescription of the upper lateral incisor favours palatal root torque. To address this, the lateral incisor bracket can be inverted. The effect of this is to change the torque prescription of the bracket to promote labial movement of the root.

In terms of numeric values, mandibular premolar brackets typically have the highest torque prescription (of up to 22°). Consequently, where significant torque differential is required, these can be particularly useful on teeth with curved surfaces (Fig. 3.6u–x).

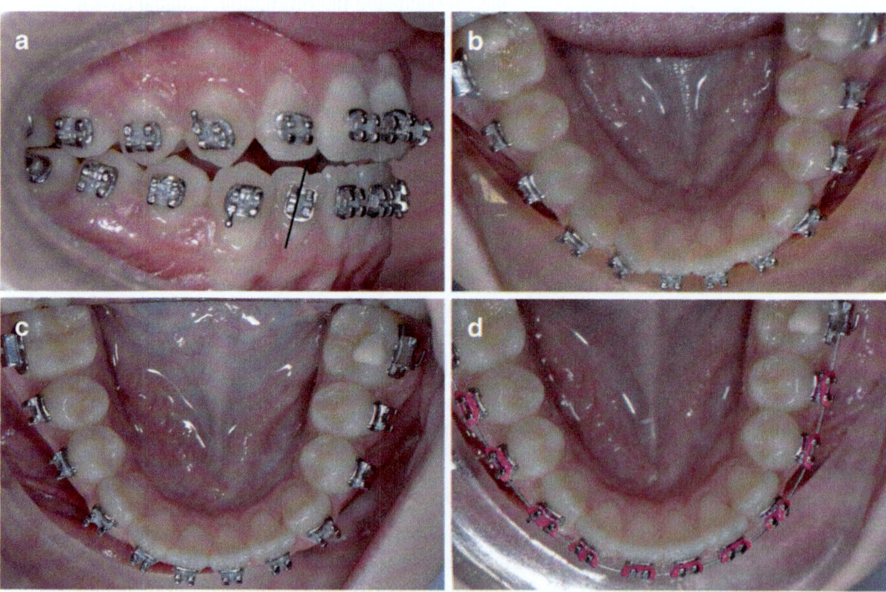

Fig. 3.6 (**a–d**) Due to the rotation, positioning the LR2 bracket in the optimal position will impede full ligation of the initial lower 0.014-in. Nickel-Titanium archwire. The LR2 bracket is placed mesial to both the centre of the clinical crown and long axis of the tooth to allow full archwire ligation into the bracket slot (**a**, **b**). At the following treatment visit, the LR2 has been derotated allowing better access to the centre of the clinical crown (**c**). The LR2 bracket is repositioned into the ideal position, and a lower 0.014-in. Nickel-Titanium archwire is religated, allowing complete rotational correction (**d**)

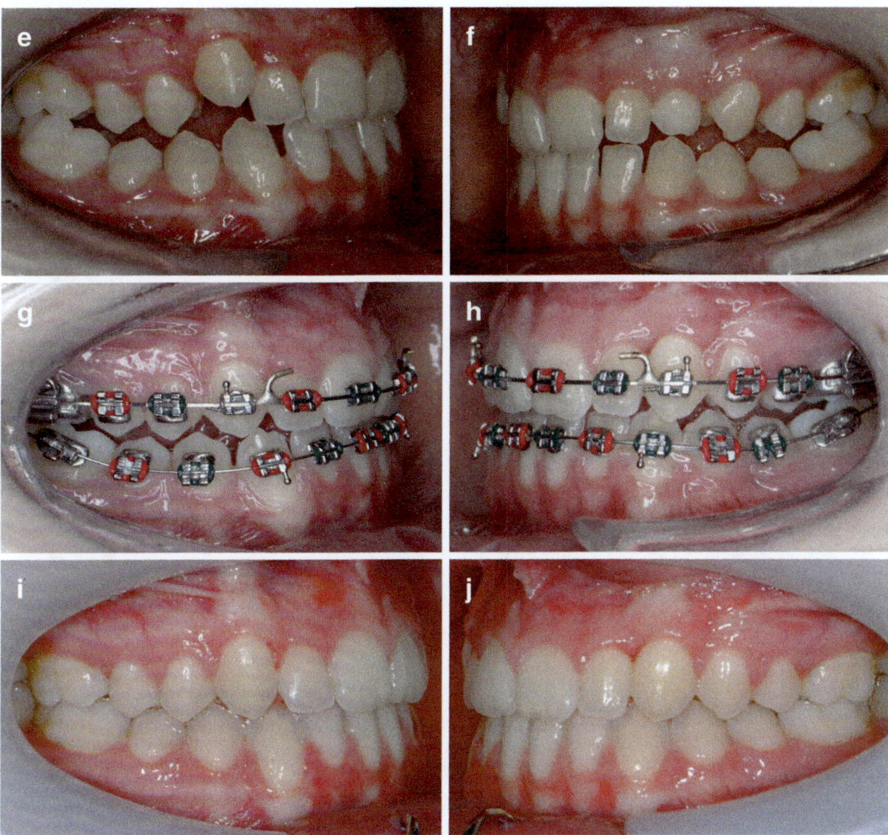

Fig. 3.6 (continued) (**e**–**j**) A Class III malocclusion exhibiting dental compensation within the lower arch with retroclined mandibular incisors and distally angulated LR3 and LL3 (**e**, **f**). The treatment plan involved levelling and alignment of the upper and lower arches on a non-extraction basis. Contralateral mandibular canine brackets have been placed on the LR3 and LL3. The ends of the initial lower 0.014-in. Nickel-Titanium archwire have also been cinched back. The aim of these treatment mechanics is to maintain the arch length, the distal canine crown angulation and both positive overjet and overbite. A positive overjet and overbite were maintained (**i**, **j**)

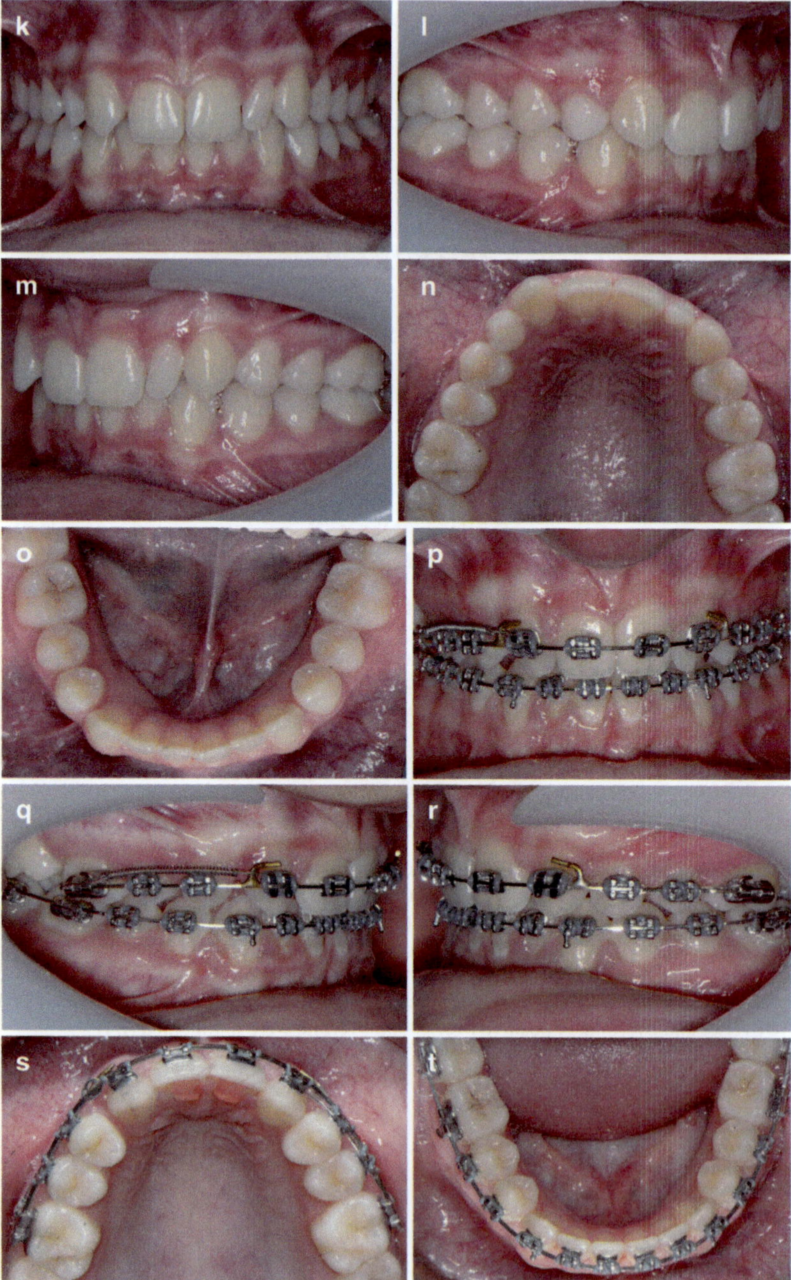

Fig. 3.6 (continued) (**k**–**t**) A Class I incisor relationship with developmental absence of the maxillary right lateral incisor. A decision was made to substitute the maxillary canines for the lateral incisors (**k**–**o**). The maxillary canine brackets were inverted (with Andrews prescription) in order to promote additional (7°) palatal root torque to better simulate the appearance of lateral incisors (**p**–**t**). Space closure in the maxillary arch would necessitate preferential posterior movement of the maxillary posterior segments; therefore, mandibular incisor advancement and lower arch lengthening would be unhelpful complicating space closure in the maxillary arch. The mandibular canine brackets were reversed to avoid arch lengthening facilitating space closure in the maxillary arch treating to Class II molar relationships bilaterally.

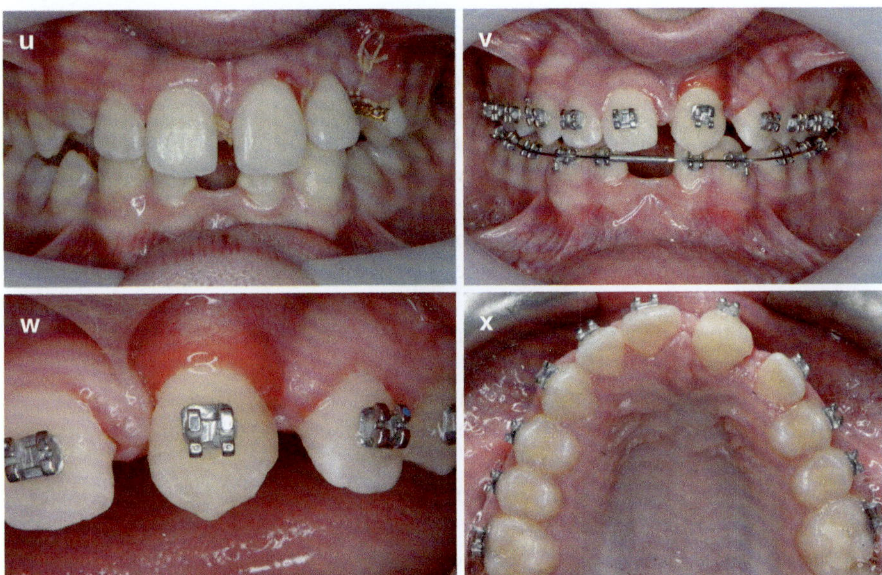

Fig. 3.6 (continued) (**u**–**x**) An 11-year-old male presented with a complex Class II division 1 incisor relationship with missing mandibular central incisors and an ectopic maxillary left canine (**u**–**x**). The canine induced significant external root resorption on the adjacent central incisor and a decision was made to substitute the canine for the incisor (**u**). Mechanical eruption was carried out with elastomeric chain to a relatively rigid (0.018-in.) stainless steel wire before using a flexible (0.014-in.) NiTi piggyback wire to achieve vertical movement of the canine as the latter has a large anchorage value and is therefore likely to lead to reactive intrusion of neighbouring teeth as it is extruded. As the canine root was buccally placed, a significant amount of palatal root torque was required to correct the root position and improve the inclination of the crown. An inverted mandibular second premolar bracket was therefore placed (with 22° of palatal root torque) with torque expression occurring in rectangular wires (**v**–**x**). The lower second premolar bracket is suitable in view of the ample numeric torque value but also its curved shape ensuring acceptable adaptation to the canine

Box 3.3 Orthodontic Bonding to Enamel Surfaces

Following etching of the enamel surface with 37% phosphoric acid and application of primer (hydroxyethylmethacrylate), an adhesive layer promotes micromechanical bonding between the enamel surface and the base of the bracket onto the tooth surface. Two techniques, one-stage (self-etching primer; Fig. 3.7) or two-stage (acid-etch and primer; Fig. 3.8), are commonly used to prepare the enamel surface prior to bonding the bracket. The single-stage (self-etching primer) technique is particularly technique-sensitive, and manufacturers' instructions should be closely followed. Enamel surface cleaning with pumice prior to application of self-etching primer is advocated (Burgess et al. 2006). However, although clinically time-efficient, a higher rate of bond failures over a 12-month period has been reported with one-stage (self-etch) compared to two-stage (acid-etch and primer) techniques (Fleming et al. 2012).

Orthodontic brackets and buccal molar tubes are available pre-coated with a layer of composite adhesive on the base of the bracket (Fig. 3.9a–e). Conventionally, however, brackets are not pre-coated and hence require direct placement of a layer of composite adhesive onto the bracket base (Fig. 3.10a–c). No significant differences in bond failures have been reported in clinical research over a 6-month period with these approaches (Wong and Power 2003).

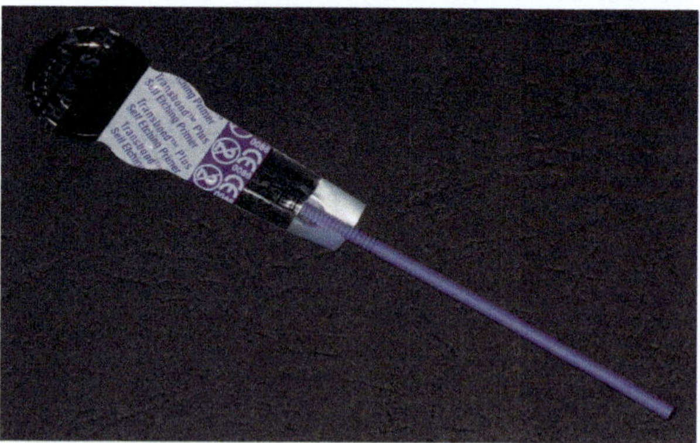

Fig. 3.7 Self-etching primer

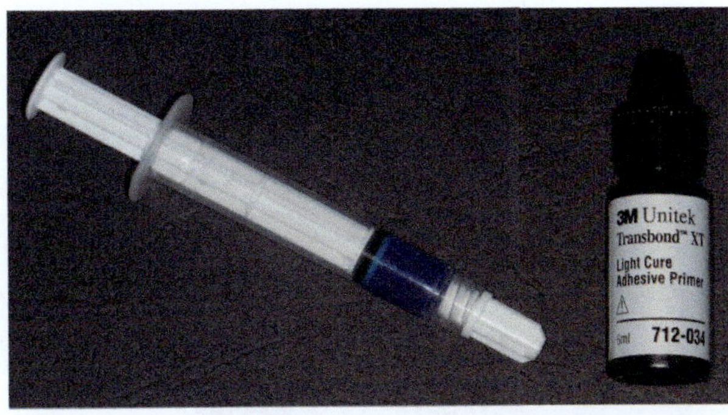

Fig. 3.8 37% phosphoric acid-etch and bonding agent

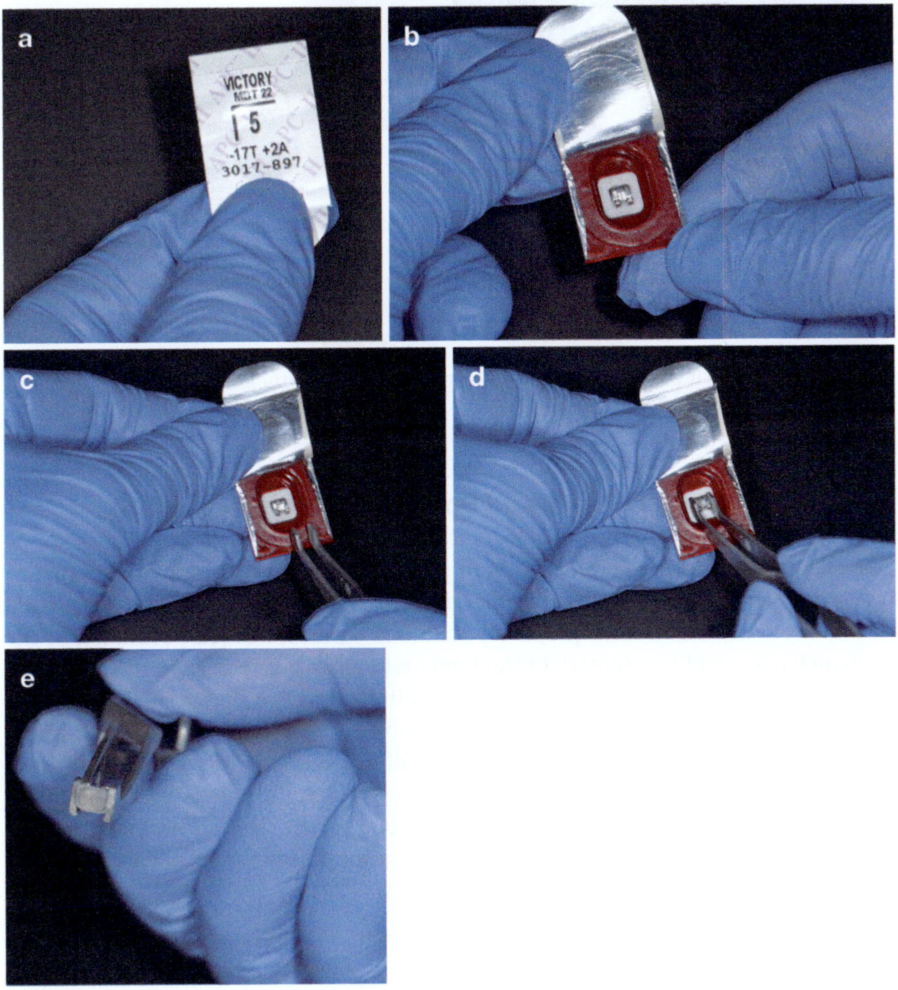

Fig. 3.9 (**a**–**e**) Pre-coated brackets allowing standardization of adhesive coating and reducing the need for chairside assistance

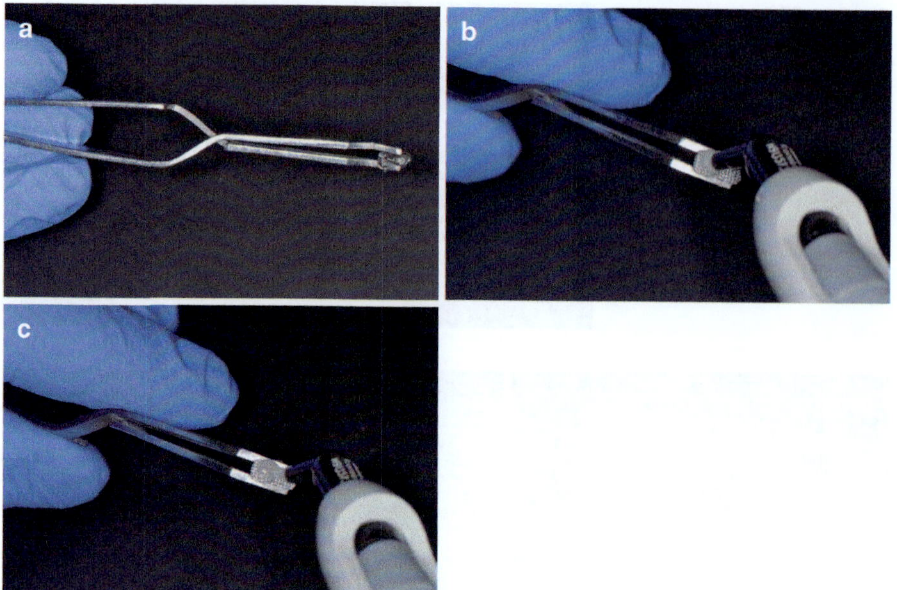

Fig. 3.10 (a–c) Uncoated molar attachments requiring placement of a layer of adhesive material

The practical steps involved in placing orthodontic brackets and bands are outlined below.

3.1 Bracket Placement and Positioning: Practical Steps

The enamel surface can be cleaned with pumice to remove any potential contaminants and salivary pellicle that could affect the achievement of adequate bond strengths (Fig. 3.11). Before preparing the tooth surface, adequate isolation of the teeth and a dry field is essential. Orthodontic retractors can be used to move the lips and cheeks away from the surface of the teeth to improve both visualisation and access to the teeth (Fig. 3.12a–c). Saliva ejectors are useful in ensuring a dry field and also prop open the occlusion (Fig. 3.13) allowing access to assess mesio-distal positioning with a mirror from the occlusal perspective. It is sensible to place the ejector in the molar region once the teeth have been dried. This allows more significant disclusion than siting in the incisal region affording room for placement of the mirror to define bracket position.

For the two-stage (acid-etch and primer) bonding technique, 37% phosphoric acid is initially placed on the teeth for 15 s (Fig. 3.14a). For molar teeth, 30 s is advised (Johnston et al. 1998) with no further advantage associated with etch times of up to 60 s. The etch is then washed from the teeth and air-dried using a 3-in-1 (Fig. 3.14b). Washing can be undertaken in one continuous 'sweep' with high-volume suction being used in the same motion to avoid accumulation of excess water and unwanted dispersal of etchant material, particularly on the soft tissues. The enamel surface should develop a "frosted" appearance (Fig. 3.14c). A thin layer of primer (hydroxyethylmethacrylate, Transbond™ XT light cure adhesive primer, 3M Unitek) is then applied to the surface of the teeth; this may be light-cured (Fig. 3.14d).

If a one-stage (self-etching primer (Transbond Plus, 3M Unitek)) technique is being employed, the surface of the teeth does not need to be prepared with 37% phosphoric acid as the etching and application of the bonding agent are combined. The self-etch primer is sequentially activated leaving a yellowish fluid at the end of the microbrush (Fig. 3.15a–f). The surface of the tooth should be agitated with the brush for 3–5 s and then lightly air-dried (Fig. 3.15g).

Using a bracket tweezers, the orthodontic bracket or molar tube with composite adhesive on the base is seated onto the tooth surface (Fig. 3.16a–c). The position of the bracket or molar tube can be adjusted using a short probe (Fig. 3.16d, e). Bracket positioning can be assessed from the labial aspect for vertical and horizontal position (relative to the centre of the clinical crown) either directly for the upper anteriors or using a dental mirror for the posterior teeth and viewed occlusally to evaluate position in relation to the long axis of the tooth (Fig. 3.16f, g). Once optimal bracket or molar tube position is achieved, full seating can be ensured either with the bracket tweezer or short probe expelling residual composite to obtain an even layer of adhesive beneath the bracket base. Residual composite flash should be removed from around the bracket base using a short probe to avoid potential plaque-harbouring areas (Fig. 3.16h, i).

The composite beneath the bracket is then light-cured with either a light-emitting diode, halogen or plasma arc laser light cure initiating the polymerisation process for the time recommended by the manufacturer. Curing times tend to be shorter for plasma arc lights, although no difference in bond failure rates has been shown between the various approaches (Fleming et al. 2013).

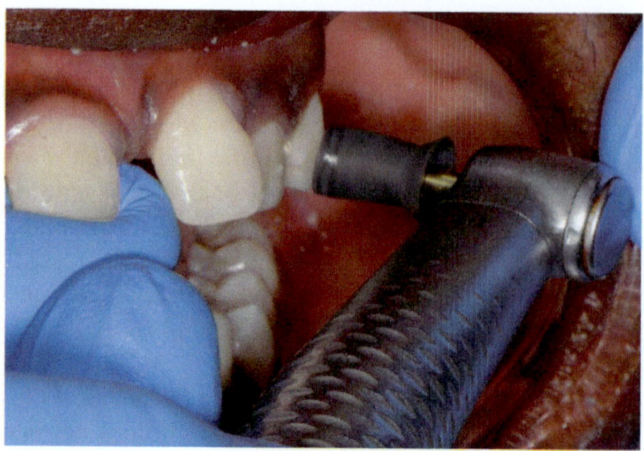

Fig. 3.11 Cleaning of the enamel surface with pumice to remove surface contaminants

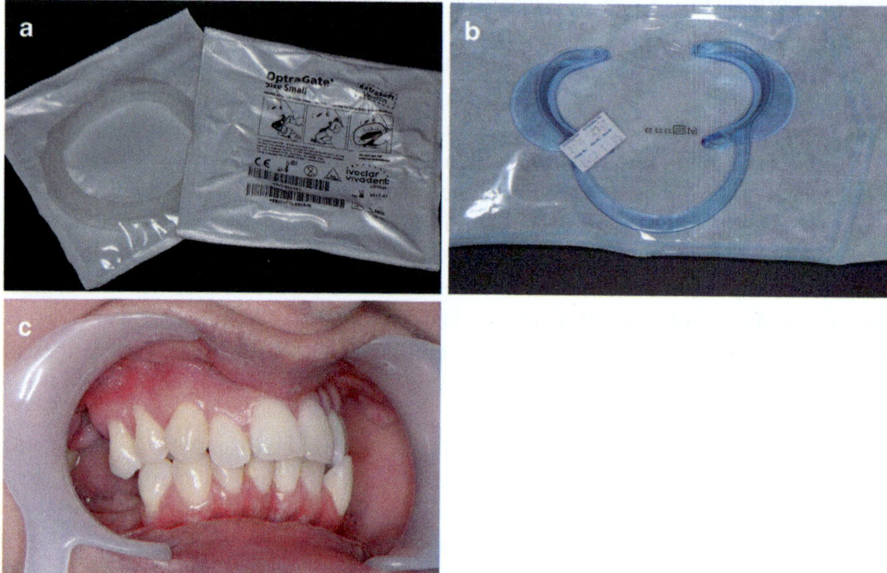

Fig. 3.12 (**a**–**c**) Disposable (**a**) and non-disposable plastic (**b**, **c**) cheek retractors to improve visual and physical access for bonding

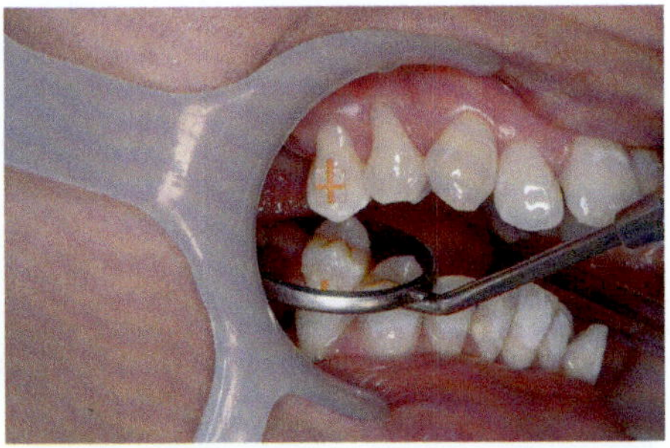

Fig. 3.13 A saliva ejector has been placed in the left second molar region allowing placement of a mouth mirror to guide mesio-distal bracket position on the maxillary right second premolar

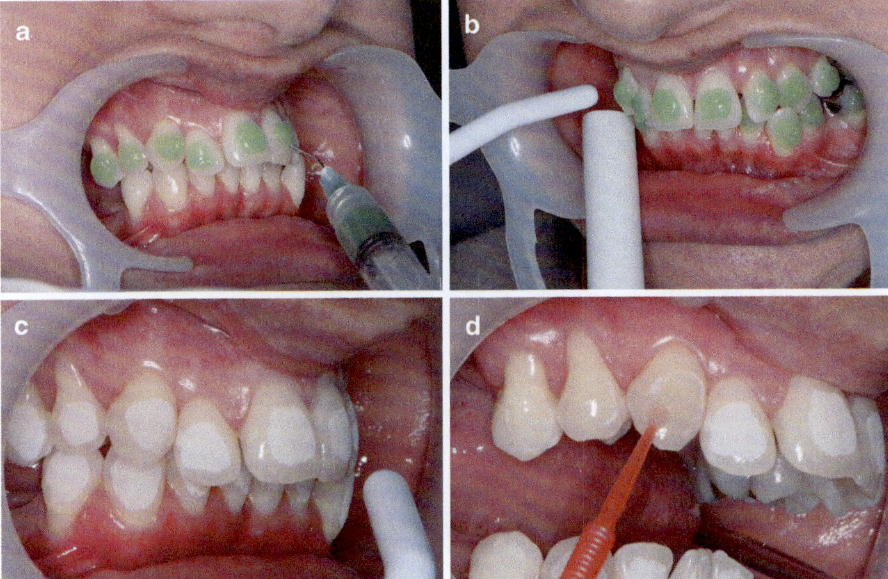

Fig. 3.14 (**a–d**) Acid etch (**a**), which is washed away under high-volume suction (**b**) leaving a frosted surface (**c**) prior to placement of bonding agent (**d**)

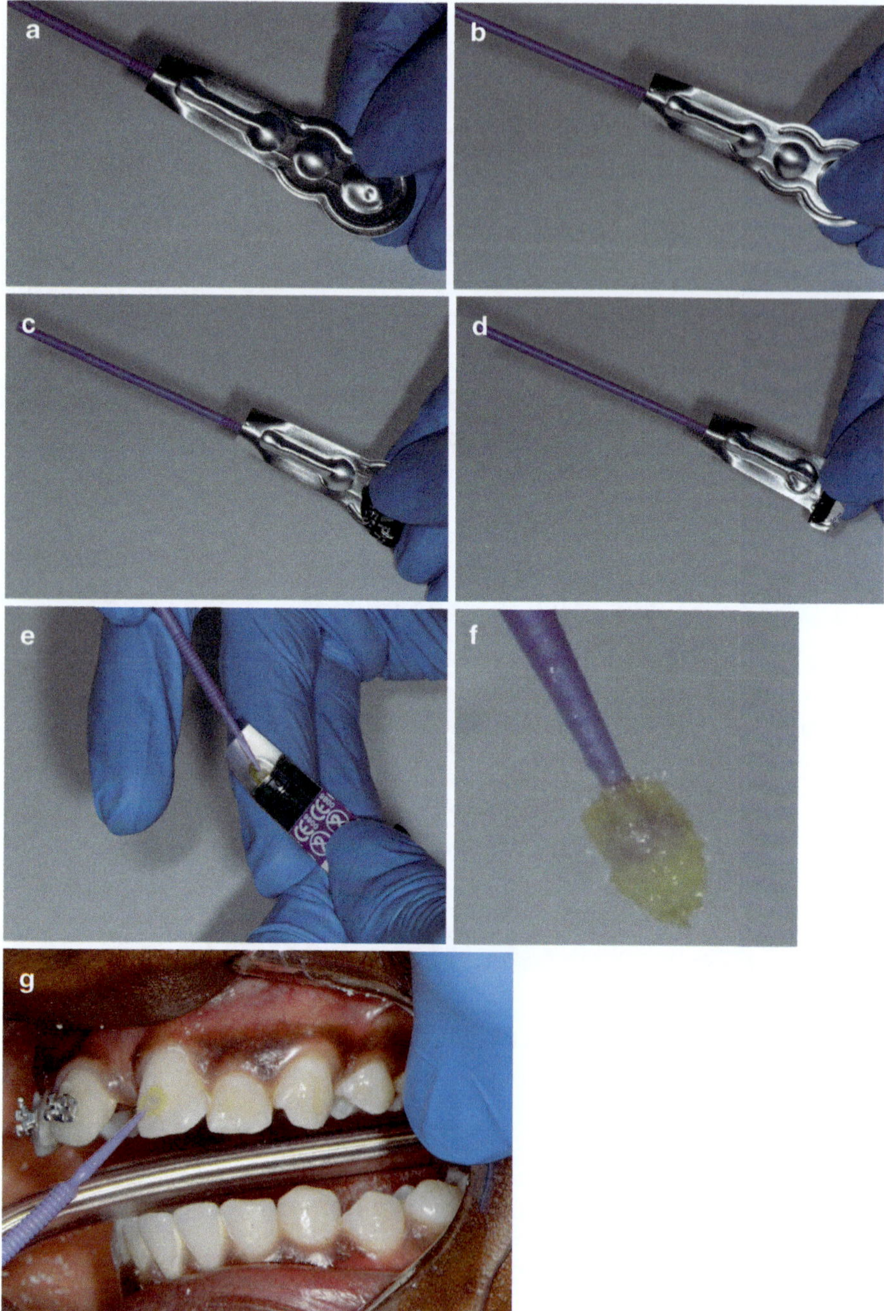

Fig. 3.15 (**a**–**g**) A one-stage technique with activation of the self-etch primer producing a yellowish fluid which is agitated on the enamel surface for 3 to 5 seconds before light air-drying

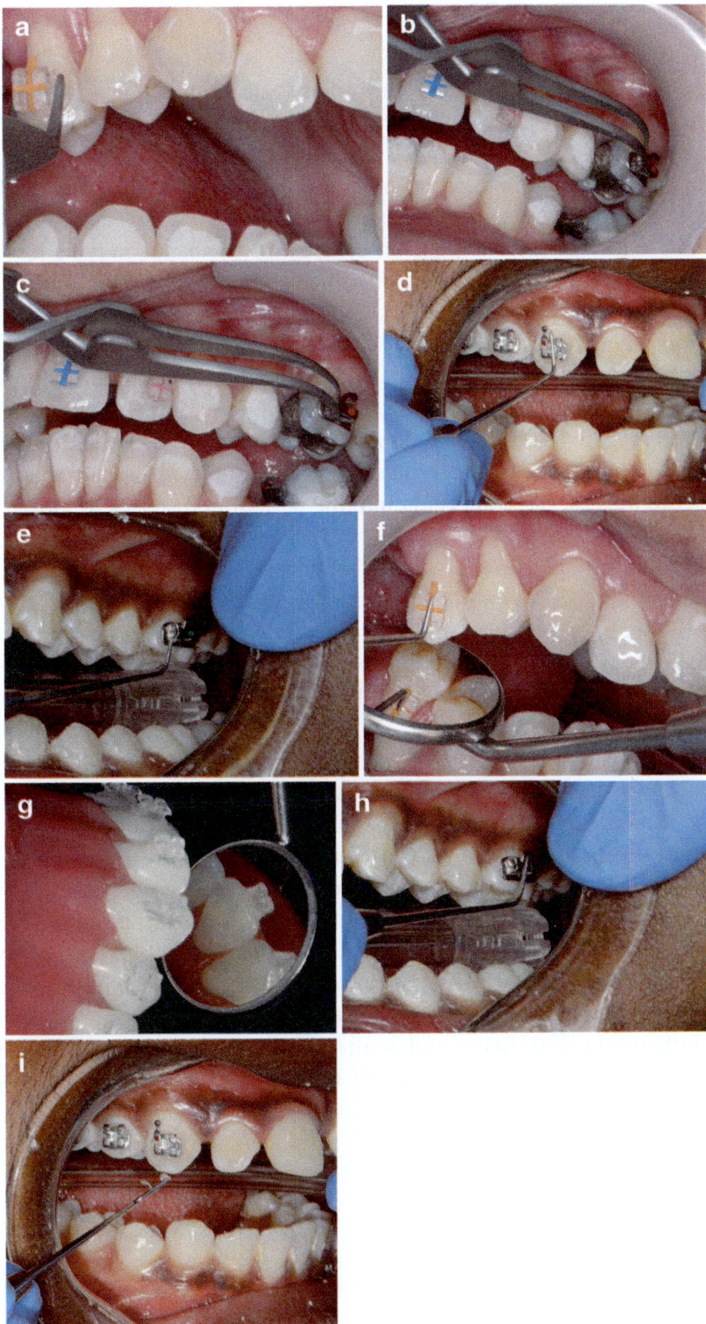

Fig. 3.16 (**a**–**i**) Bracket and molar tube positioning using a short probe with positive pressure to expel excess adhesive material and use of a saliva ejector to facilitate accurate positioning using a dental mirror

3.2 Banding of Molar Teeth

Two types of attachments are used on molar teeth: bands (Fig. 3.17a) or buccal tubes (Fig. 3.17b). The latter have become increasingly popular (and preferred by the authors) due to the ability to position these predictably, their simplicity and requirement for fewer appointments and associated comfort. However, molar bands are versatile and can be used in the construction of auxiliary appliances such as transpalatal arches and fixed expansion devices. Molar bands may be less prone to failure than molar tubes and hence can be utilised in cases where repeated buccal molar tube failures occur (Nazir et al. 2011; Millett et al. 2017), particularly on heavily-restored or misshapen teeth.

A week before molar bands are fitted, separators are placed between the mesial and distal contact points of the tooth to be banded. Elastomeric separators are usually preferred (Fig. 3.18a) to metal alternatives being simple to place and providing sufficient space (Hoffman 1972). Separators should not be left longer than this timeframe to avoid the risk of submerging into the periodontal spaces or falling out. The aim of separation is to provide at least 0.3 mm space (Cureton and Bice 1997) between the adjacent teeth, to allow comfortable seating and placement of the band. Separators can be placed using dental floss (Fig. 3.18b–f), using two mosquito forceps (Fig. 3.18g, h) or a bespoke plier. Irrespective of the technique, the separator is stretched and gently seated above and below the contact point between the teeth (Fig. 3.18i, j). Following the placement of separators, tenderness and discomfort are commonplace and typically more severe than following fixed appliance placement or adjustment (Ngan et al. 1989).

Various band sizes can be selected. Fit can first be gauged on physical study models to assess the required size before being tested on the tooth limiting inventory requirements. Initially, the band can be located onto the tooth using fingers (Fig. 3.19a, b) before being passed through the contact points by applying gentle pressure in a gingival direction using a Mershon band pusher (Chap. 2) (Fig. 3.19c–e). Ideally, the band should be adapted as closely as possible to the surface of the tooth. For maxillary molar bonds, the tube should lie adjacent to the buccal groove (Fig. 3.19f). From the buccal aspect, the band should be parallel with the buccal cusps and with even amount of the mesial and distal cusps visible (Fig. 3.19g). Care should be taken to avoid over-seating of the band, particularly palatally. The slot of the mandibular first molar bands should be positioned onto the mesio-buccal groove of the tooth, and similar to upper molars, the buccal aspect of the band should usually be parallel with the buccal cusps and an even amount of the mesial and distal cusps visible from the buccal aspect.

Once the correct size band has been chosen, it should be removed from the molar tooth using posterior band remover pliers (see Chap. 10) and cleaned. For cementation, a layer of glass polyalkenoate cement (glass ionomer luting cement; Ketac™ Cem radiopaque 3M ESPE) can be applied to the inner aspect of the band with a flat plastic instrument (Fig. 3.19h–k). The cement should chemically adhere the band to the enamel but also occupy the void between the band and the tooth surface, thus increasing mechanical retention. Once fitted to the tooth and prior to setting of the cement, the tooth/band can be cleaned with a moist cotton wool roll with air blown through the buccal tube to remove any residue, which might otherwise impede wire insertion if this is allowed to set.

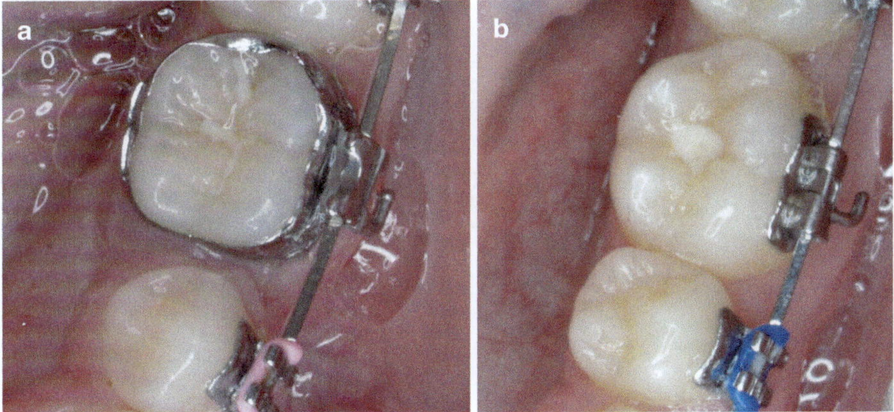

Fig. 3.17 (**a**, **b**) Banding (**a**) and bracketing (**b**) of mandibular first molars. While bonded attachments (**b**) simplify attachment placement and streamline patient care, there is limited evidence of associated benefit in terms of attachment failure and periodontal health

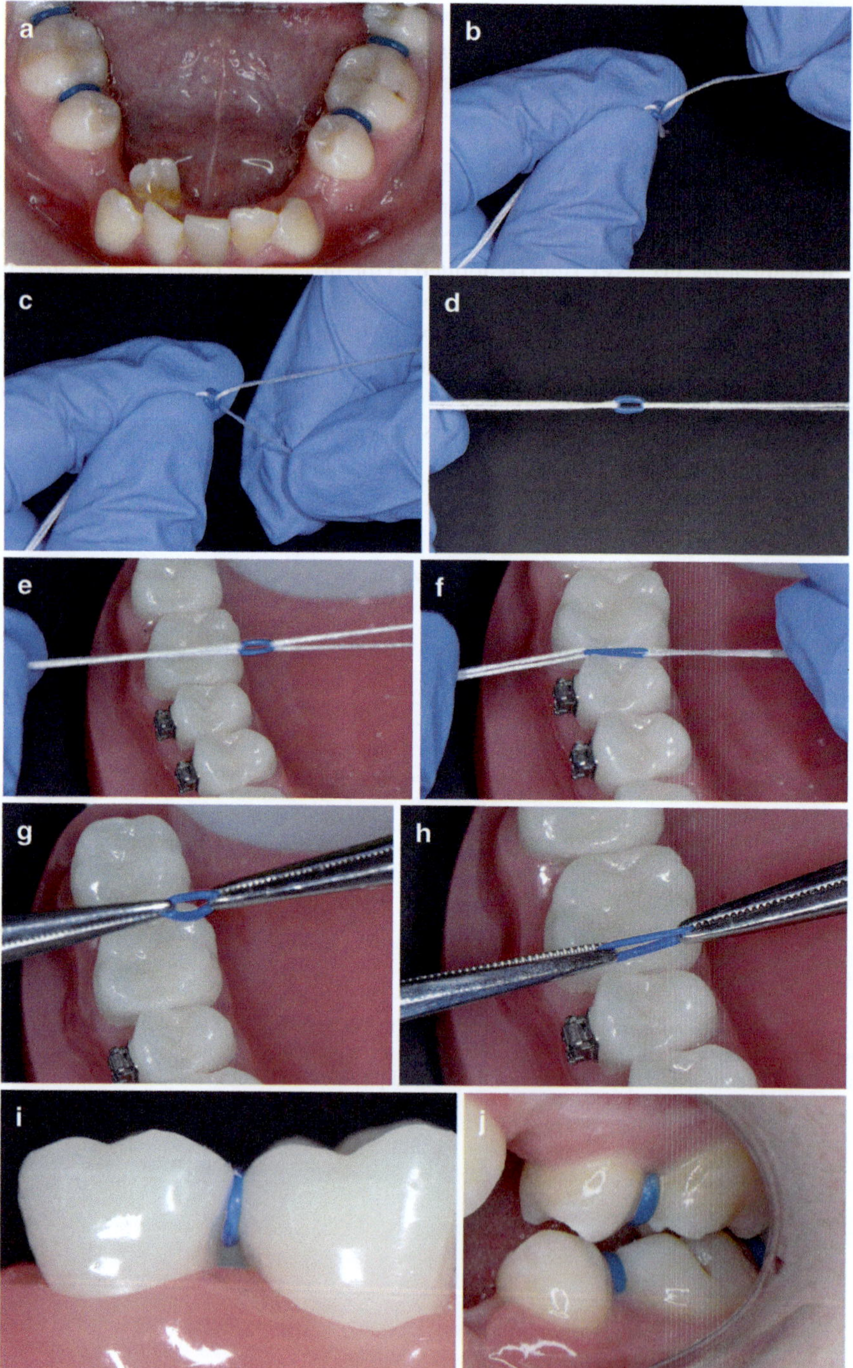

Fig. 3.18 (**a**–**j**) Elastomeric separators can be placed either with dental floss, a pair of mosquito forceps (**g**, **h**) or bespoke pliers

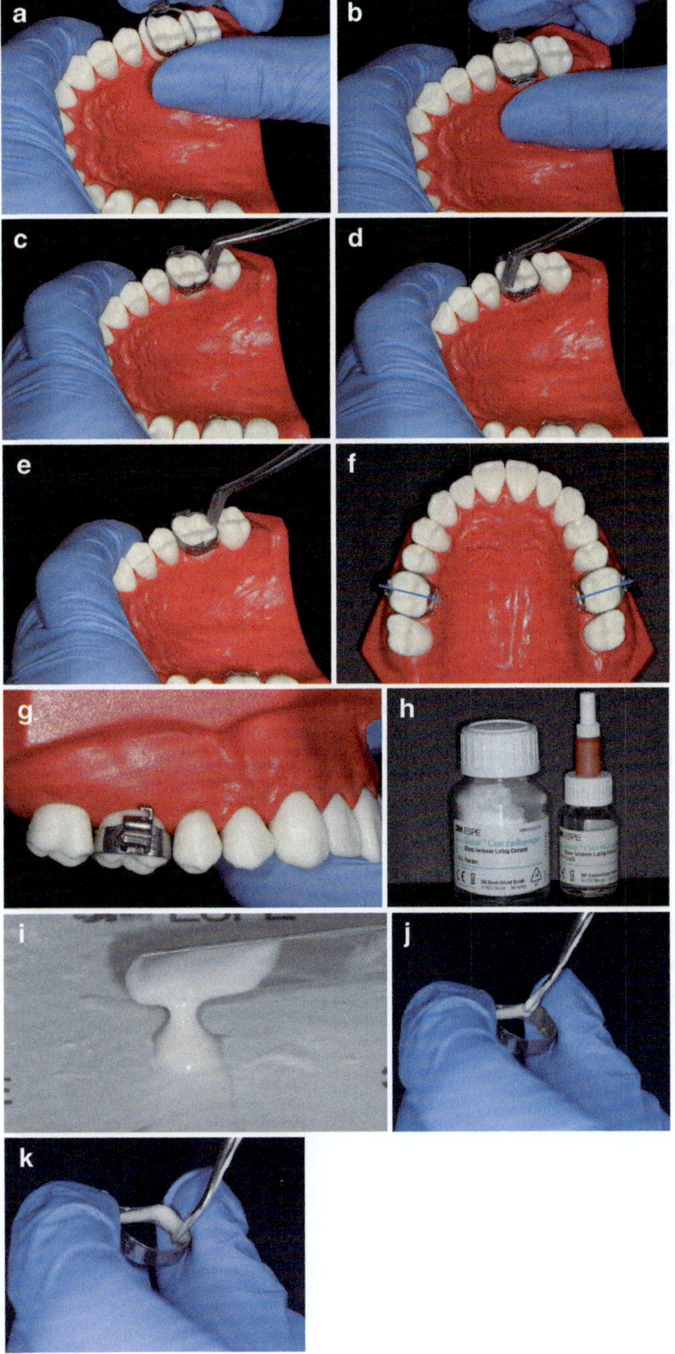

Fig. 3.19 (**a–k**) Band placement on the maxillary molar using a Mershon band pusher (**e**). Care should be taken to avoid over-seating particularly palatally

References

Armstrong D, Shen G, Petocz P, Darendeliler MA. A comparison of accuracy in bracket positioning between two techniques—localizing the centre of the clinical crown and measuring the distance from the incisal edge. Eur J Orthod. 2007;29(5):430–6.

Buonocore MG. A simple method of increasing the adhesion of acrylic filling materials to enamel surfaces. J Dent Res. 1955;34(6):849–53.

Burgess AM, Sherriff M, Ireland AJ. Self-etching primers: is prophylactic pumicing necessary? A randomized clinical trial. Angle Orthod. 2006;76(1):114–8.

Carlson SK, Johnson E. Bracket positioning and resets: five steps to align crowns and roots consistently. Am J Orthod Dentofac Orthop. 2001;119(1):76–80.

Cureton S, Bice RW. Comparison of three types of separators in adult patients. J Clin Orthod. 1997;31(3):172–7.

Fleming PS, Johal A, Pandis N. Self-etch primers and conventional acid-etch technique for orthodontic bonding: a systematic review and meta-analysis. Am J Orthod Dentofac Orthop. 2012;142(1):83–94.

Fleming PS, Eliades T, Katsaros C, Pandis N. Curing lights for orthodontic bonding: a systematic review and meta-analysis. Am J Orthod Dentofac Orthop. 2013;143(4 Suppl):S92–103.

Hoffman WE. A study of four types of separators. Am J Orthod Dentofac Orthop. 1972;62(1):67–73.

Johnston CD, Burden DJ, Hussey DL, Mitchell CA. Bonding to molars—the effect of etch time (an in vitro study). Eur J Orthod. 1998;20(2):195–9.

McLaughlin RP, Bennett JC, Trevisi HJ. Systemized orthodontic treatment mechanics. St. Louis: Elsevier Health Sciences; 2001.

Millett DT, Mandall NA, Mattick RC, Hickman J, Glenny AM. Adhesives for bonded molar tubes during fixed brace treatment. Cochrane Database Syst Rev. 2017;2:CD008236.

Nazir M, Walsh T, Mandall NA, Matthew S, Fox D. Banding versus bonding of first permanent molars: a multi-centre randomized controlled trial. J Orthod. 2011;38(2):81–9.

Ngan P, Kess B, Wilson S. Perception of discomfort by patients undergoing orthodontic treatment. Am J Orthod Dentofac Orthop. 1989;96(1):47–53.

Reynolds IR, von Fraunhofer JA. Direct bonding of orthodontic attachments to teeth: the relation of adhesive bond strength to gauze mesh size. Br J Orthod. 1976;3(3):91–5.

Silveira GS, de Almeida NV, Pereira DM, Mattos CT, Mucha JN. Prosthetic replacement vs space closure for maxillary lateral incisor agenesis: a systematic review. Am J Orthod Dentofac Orthop. 2016;150(2):228–37.

Taylor NG, Cook PA. The reliability of positioning pre-adjusted brackets: an in vitro study. Br J Orthod. 1992;19(1):25–34.

Wong M, Power S. A prospective randomized clinical trial to compare pre-coated and non-precoated brackets. J Orthod. 2003;30(2):155–8.

Initial Alignment

4

Initial orthodontic alignment typically represents the first phase of fixed appliance-based treatment. The objectives of this stage include correction of horizontal and rotational discrepancies (alignment), improvement of gross angulation and inclination issues and vertical correction (levelling) between adjacent teeth. Ultimately, this involves alignment of the bracket slots relative to each other permitting progression into larger dimension and stiffer wires at later treatment stages when other objectives such as overjet reduction and space closure can be achieved. In contemporary treatment, overbite reduction is increasingly undertaken in tandem with alignment; however, the specifics of overbite reduction will be described in Chap. 6.

Initial orthodontic alignment requires high degrees of wire flexibility permitting engagement of grossly displaced and irregular teeth, particularly with limited inter-bracket span in the lower anterior region and in areas of significant crowding. Alignment is usually undertaken over a period of approximately 6 months pending on the pre-existing space conditions and involves progression from low-dimension round (0.012- or 0.014-in.) Nickel-Titanium (NiTi) to larger dimension round (0.016-, 0.018- and 0.020-in.) and square or rectangular (0.020 × 0.020-, 0.017 × 0.025-, 0.018 × 0.025- and 0.019 × 0.025-in.) NiTi wires.

Archwires may be held in place using elastomerics, stainless steel ligatures or inbuilt mechanisms with self-ligating systems. Conventional modes of ligation, however, are limited in relation to efficiency of handling, plastic deformation, discoloration, plaque accumulation and friction. Self-ligating brackets have been developed in an attempt to address these shortcomings. Stainless steel ligatures may also be used in areas of significant rotation or displacement and when active mechanics are in use to promote rotational correction during alignment and indeed to limit unwanted rotations during sliding mechanics and space closure. The practical steps involvement in manipulation and engagement of initial aligning wires are outlined below.

P. Fleming, J. Seehra, *Fixed Orthodontic Appliances*, BDJ Clinician's Guides,
https://doi.org/10.1007/978-3-030-12165-5_4

4.1 Initial Wire Placement and Engagement: Practical Steps

The wire is initially cut to length with distal end cutters using the study model as a reference (Fig. 4.1) and centred using a midline indicator (Fig. 4.2). A small distal excess (3–7 mm) is advisable to allow for wire cinching and possibly for additional length in order to compensate for wire deflection with engagement of displaced and crowded teeth. Where cinching of distal ends is planned, a heat source can be used to facilitate this; however, alternative approaches are preferable.

Round wires are introduced using fingers to thread into the molar tubes initially (Fig. 4.3). A pliers (e.g. Weingarts) may be used to direct this but is often not required for narrow dimension wires.

A mosquito forceps is used with the tips enclosing one edge of the elastomeric while leaving the lumen exposed permitting a secure grip and engagement of the undercuts of tie-wings (Fig. 4.4a, b).

Ligation may be commenced in the anterior region to stabilise the wire initially. Ormolasts are typically used engaging all four tie-wings sequentially (Fig. 4.5a–e) in an O-configuration. It is advisable to engage a gingival tie-wing initially before proceeding to both occlusal tie-wings and finally the remaining gingival wing.

Partial ligation, figure-of-eight ties (Fig. 4.6a–h) and use of stainless steel ties (Fig 4.7a–k) can be considered with more displaced or rotated teeth. Partial ligation is likely to inhibit progression to a significantly larger wire at the subsequent visit. More complete ligation, however, promotes better alignment of the slots and therefore wire progression; this is, however, not always realistic in view of the degree of displacement or rotation.

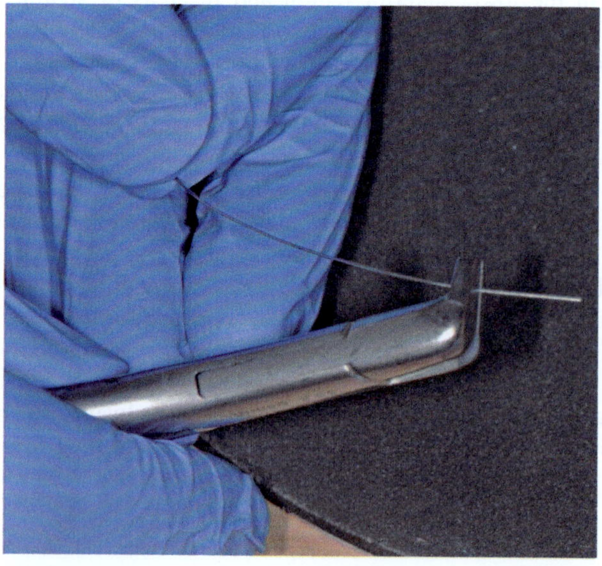

Fig. 4.1 Distal end cutter

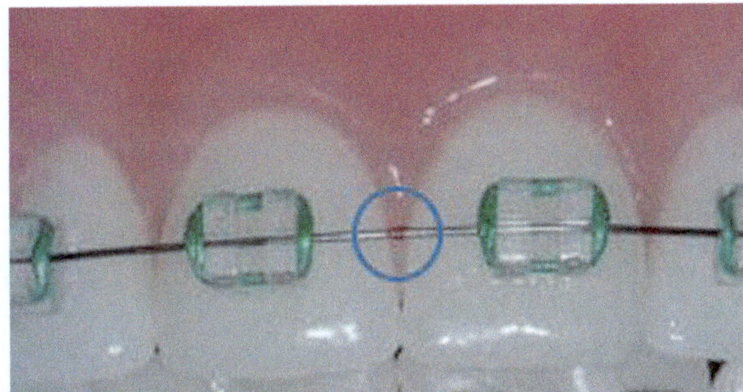

Fig. 4.2 A midline identifier (circled) on an upper 0.014-inch NiTi wire

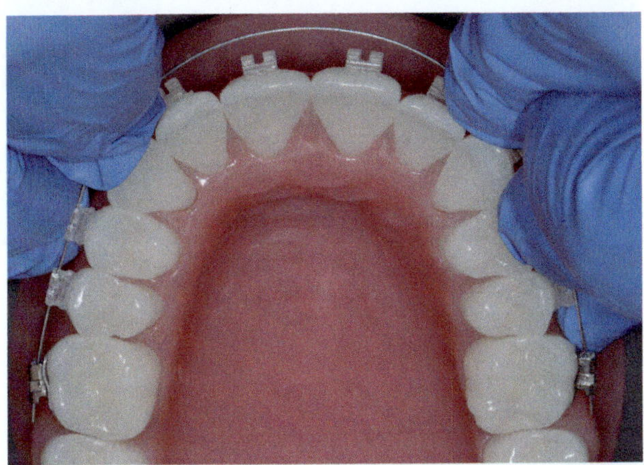

Fig. 4.3 An initial alignment NiTi wire inserted through the molar tubes using fingers only. A Weingarts may be helpful in the presence of significantly rotated molars or with larger dimension wires

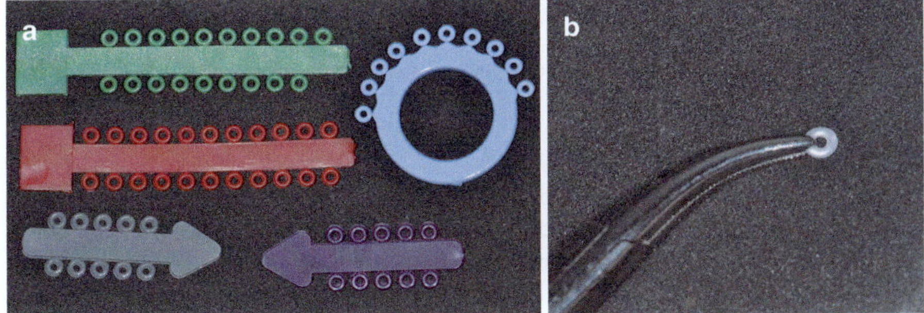

Fig. 4.4 (**a**, **b**) A range of elastomerics. (**a**) The beaks of the mosquito forceps should not encroach on the central lumen (**b**) to allow positive engagement of bracket undercuts

Pre-stretching of elastomeric (Fig. 4.6a) makes the ormolast slightly more lax permitting the degree of stretch required to allow figure-of-eight formation (Fig. 4.6b–h). Stainless steel ligatures offer potential advantages with lower resistance to sliding than elastomerics and less force decay making wire ligation more assured. Metal ties may also be used in areas of significant wire displacement. It is

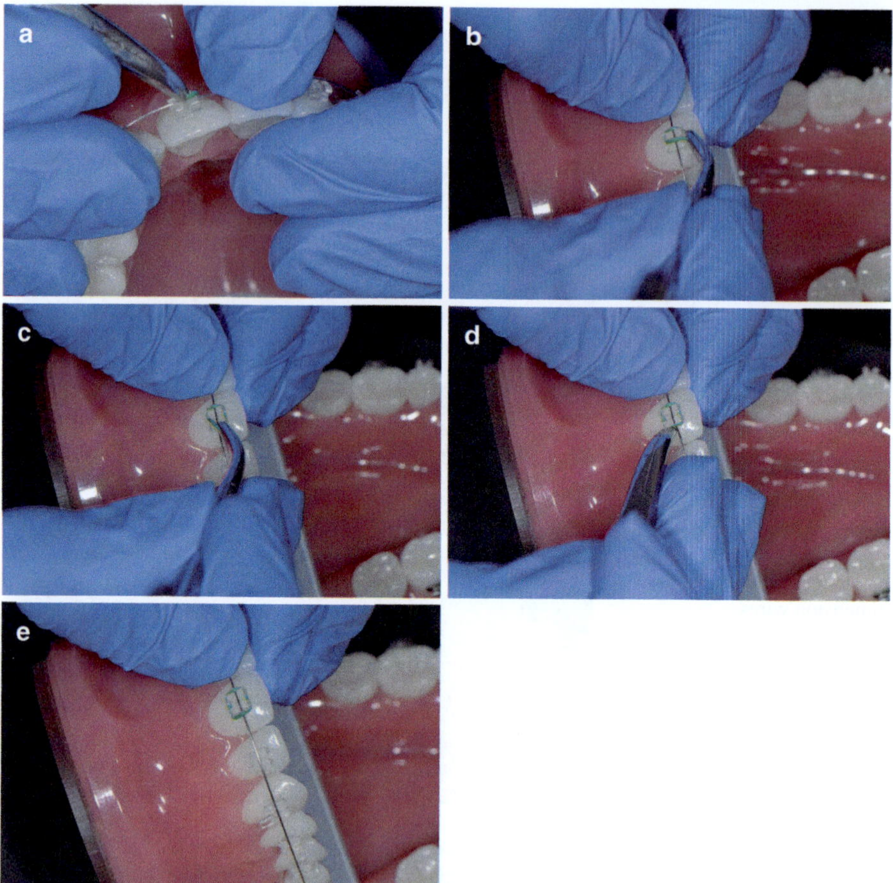

Fig. 4.5 (**a–e**) Sequential placement of an ormolast in an 'O'-configuration on the maxillary central incisor

helpful to bend the ligature at approx. 90° to assist with placement (Fig. 4.7a–d). The ligatures should ideally be tied at 90° to the plane of the bracket as shear forces on the bracket risk debonding during tightening (Fig. 4.7e–g). Similarly, the ligature cutters can be held parallel to the bracket with a wire tail of approx. 3 mm, which can be tucked occlusally with a wire tucker in order to promote optimal gingival health (Fig. 4.7h–k). Firm ligation is advised when stainless steel ligatures are used; it is important, however, that these are not over-tightened as this risks irreversible surface change to the archwire including notching, which may in turn inhibit tooth movement.

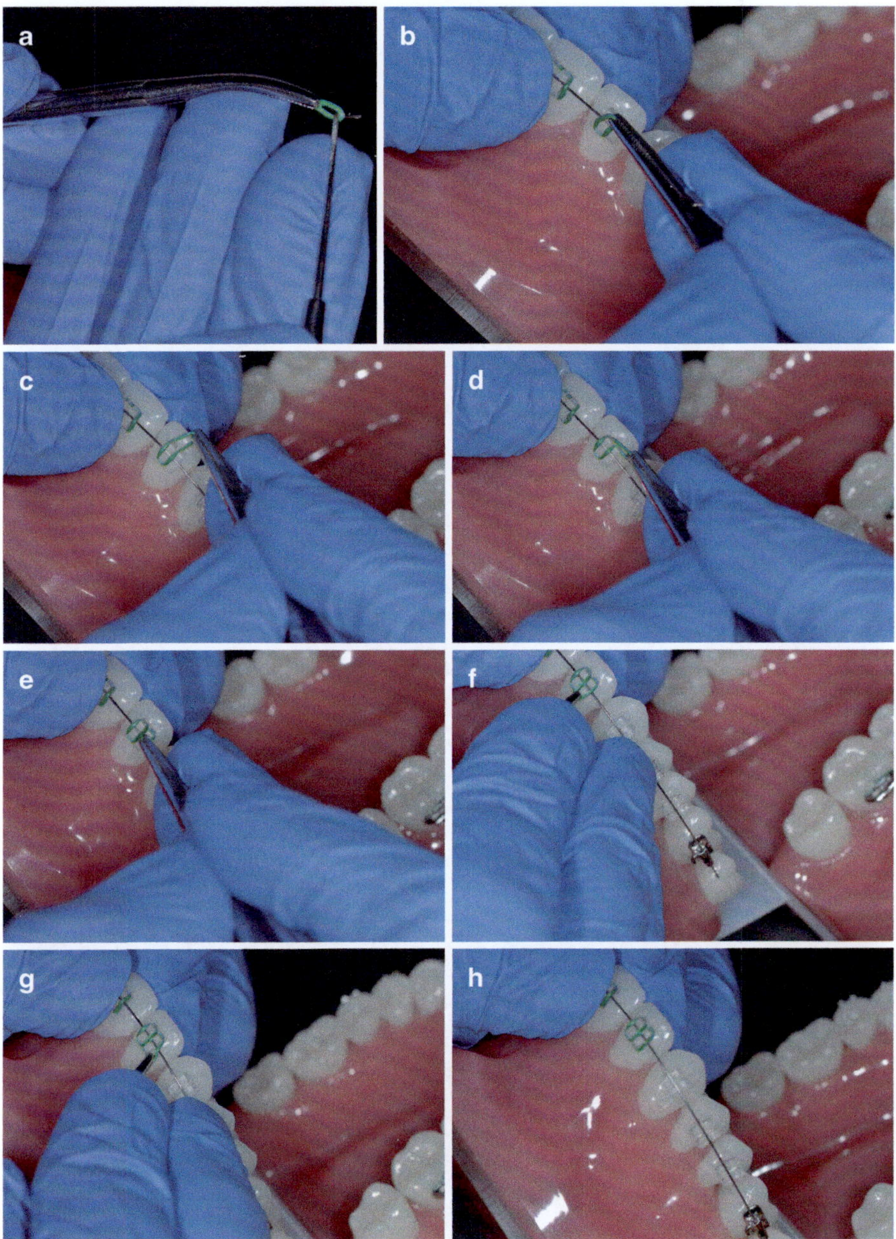

Fig. 4.6 (**a–h**) Placement of an ormolast in a figure-of-eight configuration following initial pre-stretching (**a**)

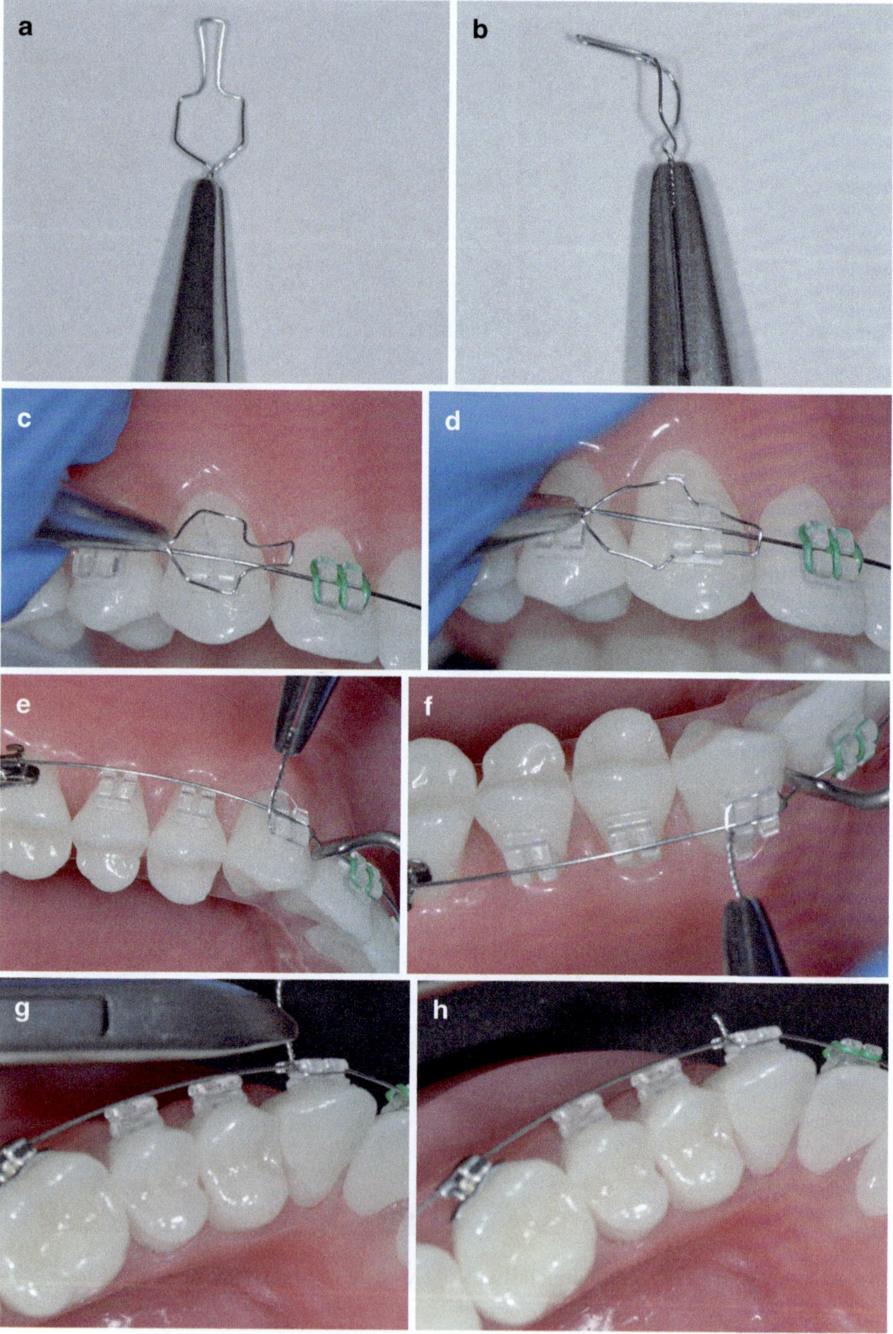

Fig. 4.7 (**a**–**k**) Placement of a stainless steel ligature. Care is taken to tie and cut the ligature at right angles to the attachment (**f**, **g**) to avoid introduction of shear forces which might predispose to attachment failure

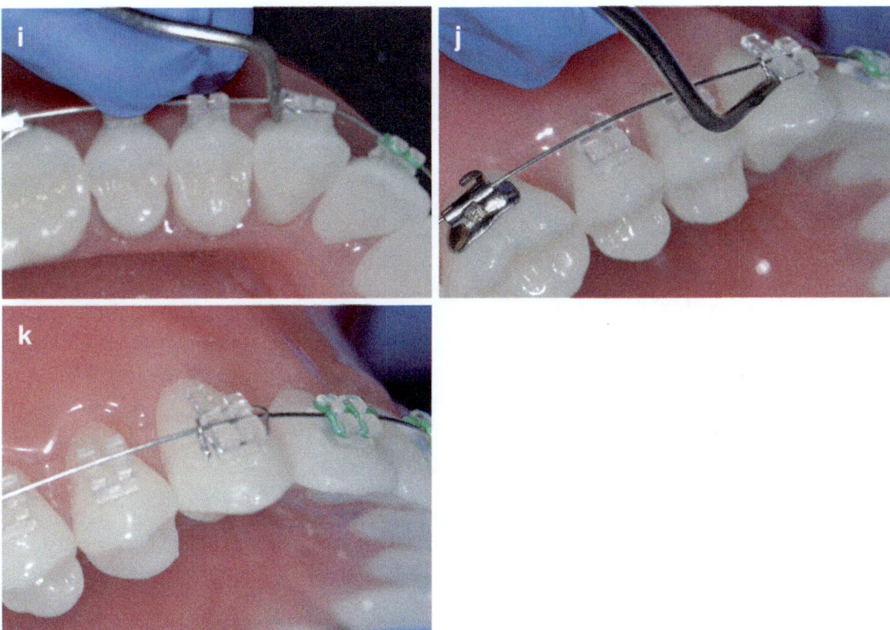

Fig. 4.7 (continued)

An initial 0.014-in. NiTi wire has been ligated (Fig. 4.8a) in this arch with significant palatal displacement of the maxillary right lateral incisor. For ease of ligation, the most displaced tooth (UR2) is ligated initially (Fig. 4.8b). This tooth can be included in the appliance at this stage as there is adequate space to allow for alignment. Where inadequate space exists, sliding mechanics and space redistribution (Chap. 5) are advisable. All teeth have been ligated fully in this case. Partial ligation can be considered where excessive wire deflection occurs as this risks excessive forces and attachment debonding. Moreover, excessive deformation may lead to the superelastic properties of the wire being exceeded.

Lacebacks have been placed bilaterally from canine to first molar (Fig. 4.9a–n). It is helpful to tie the wire off after initial engagement of the molar hook (Fig. 4.9a–j). Tie-wings of premolar and canine brackets should be engaged positively to ensure the laceback is secure (Fig. 4.9k–n). At subsequent visits, lacebacks are likely to become lax as the canines move distally and molars in a mesial direction. The laceback may be left in place, while the arch wire is removed and can be activated simply by twisting the wire with an explorer tip (Fig. 4.10).

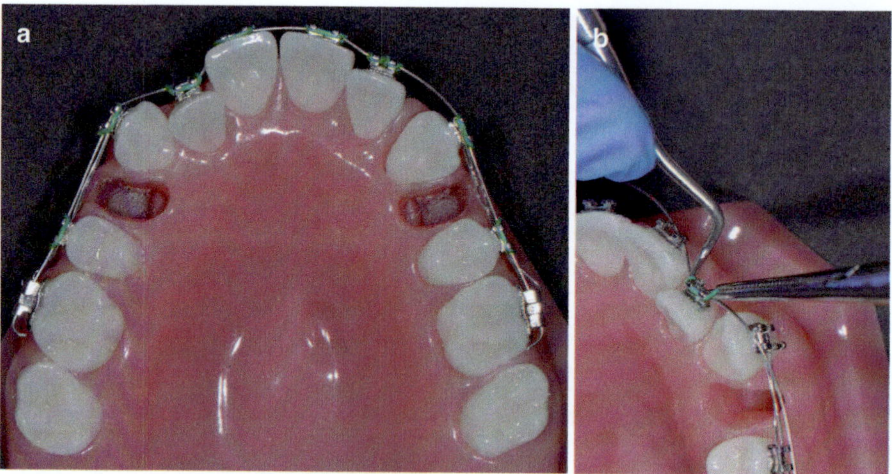

Fig. 4.8 (**a**, **b**) Engagement of a displaced maxillary lateral incisor. In this instance, there is sufficient space to align the lateral incisor (**b**); as such, sliding mechanics would be unnecessary

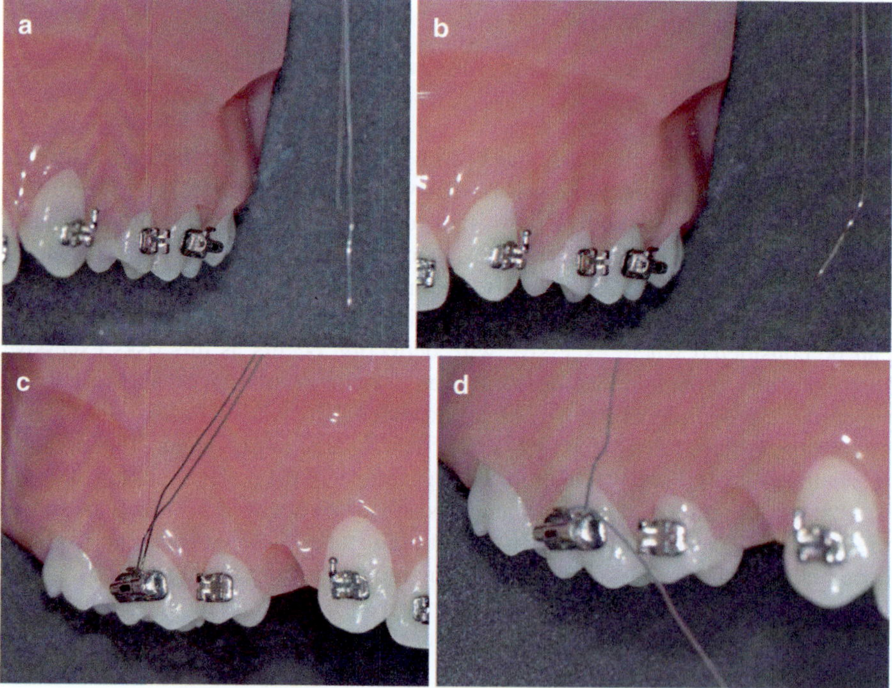

Fig. 4.9 (**a**–**n**) Placement of a laceback ligature

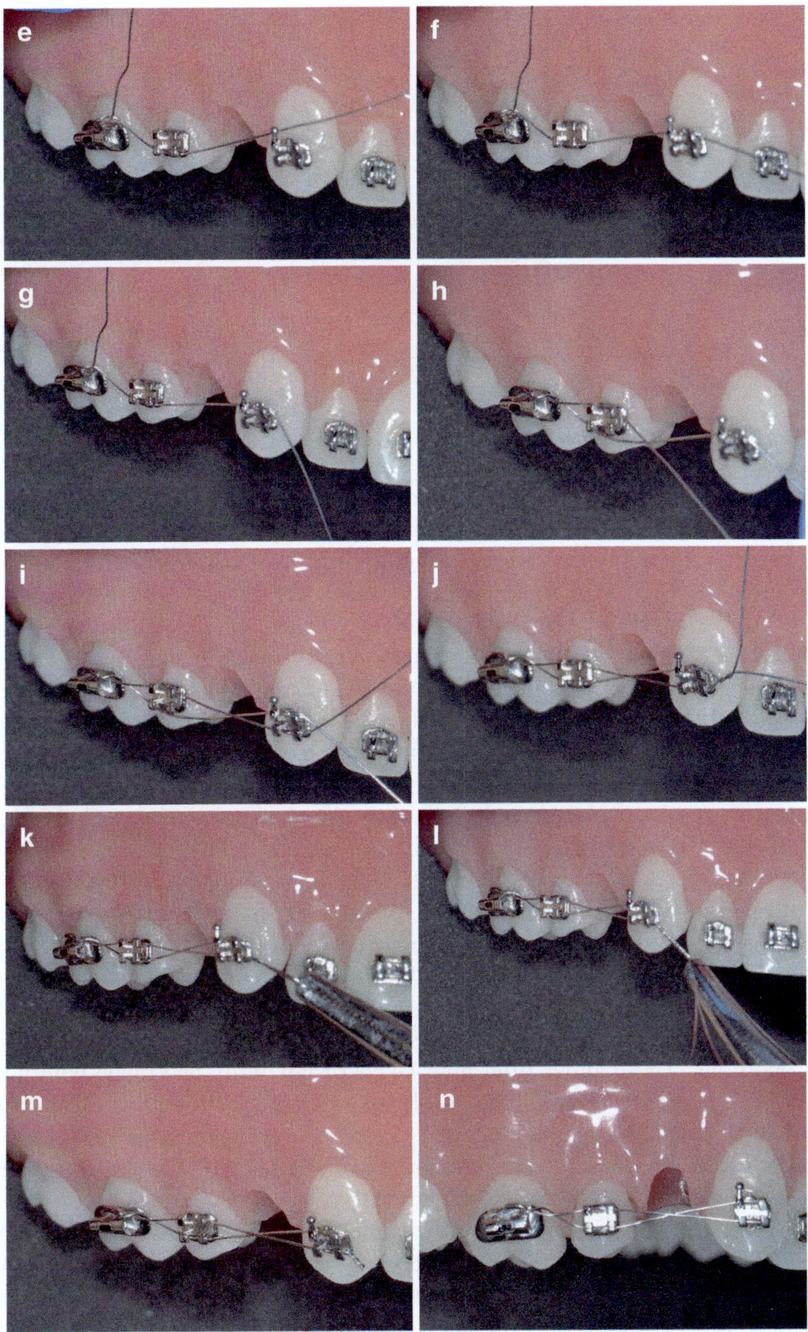

Fig. 4.9 (continued)

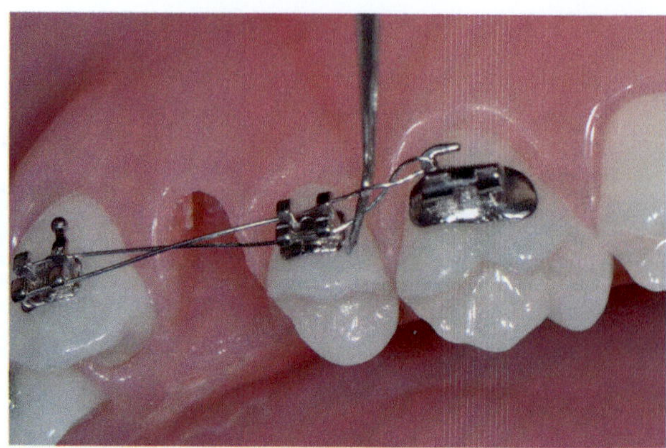

Fig. 4.10 Reactivation of a laceback using an explorer tip. This does not necessitate removal and replacement of the wire

Box 4.1 Ideal Properties of Initial Alignment Wire

Kusy (1997) has summarised the requirements of an initial aligning wire in relation to three main aspects: strength, stiffness and range. All archwires require a degree of strength in order to resist occlusal forces; however, relatively low strength is needed during the early stages of treatment with an onus on higher strength during arch levelling, overjet reduction and space closure which occur later in treatment. High range is essential early in treatment as irregularity and crowding mean that correctly positioned brackets are likely to be malaligned relative to one another in one or more spatial planes. Relatively low stiffness and high flexibility are important in order to facilitate engagement of grossly displaced teeth. Low-dimension, round NiTi wires typically fulfil these requirements. Historically, multistrand and multiloop stainless steel wires were used as alternatives to NiTi; however, these were associated with permanent deformation and increased chairside time and complexity, respectively. As such, while clinical evidence does not point to a compelling benefit of NiTi wires, they have found favour and are used almost universally as an initial aligning wire (O'Brien et al. 1990).

Nickel-titanium alloys incorporate Nickel and Titanium in relatively even proportions. These alloys offer high levels of flexibility and range with low stiffness. Moreover, second- and third-generation NiTi alloys may exhibit the added benefits of shape memory and superelastic behaviour. For orthodontic purposes, shape memory permits return to the original wire configuration over a period of intra-oral cycling. As such, with tailored, pre-formed wires, force delivery can be controlled and maintained over a sustained period. Superelasticity implies that force levels may remain constant over a range of deformation; this can be exploited in the delivery of relatively constant forces over a range of wire deflection and tooth movement. These properties rely on crystalline phase transformation induced either by stress or temperature change.

Box 4.2 Lacebacks

Lacebacks are fabricated from 0.09″ to 0.10″ stainless steel wire spanning the first molars to canines. They represent a means of controlling the anteroposterior position of the incisors during the initial alignment phase by limiting forward movement of the canine crowns while the mesial tip prescription of the canine teeth is expressed. Lacebacks are of potential value in extraction cases or spaced arches.

Orthodontic extractions may promote more stable relief of crowding by generating space to limit or avoid unwanted advancement of the anterior segments. The mesial angulation in-built in canine brackets predisposes to forward movement of the incisors in conjunction with alleviation of crowding during the initial alignment phase. While the incisors may be moved posteriorly later in treatment, particularly during space closure, reciprocal movement of this nature ('round tripping') is considered undesirable predisposing to root resorption, periodontal attachment loss and more prolonged treatment.

Lacebacks may be particularly useful where the canines are upright or distally angulated at the outset, as in these cases, significant mesial crown movement is likely to be accompanied by advancement of the incisors (Fig. 4.11a–k). Lacebacks are placed in a passive configuration and are typically intermittently activated during occlusal contact. While many clinicians routinely use lacebacks to control incisor position during orthodontic alignment, they have not met with universal approval. Disadvantages of laceback use may include loss of anchorage posteriorly manifesting as mesial migration and tipping of first permanent molars, potential for plaque stagnation and limited additional chairside time and complexity. Moreover, clinical trials have confirmed that control of incisor position comes at the expense of anchorage loss in the molar region (Irvine et al. 2004). As such, they remain useful in terms of alignment but are unlikely to alter the anchorage balance appreciably.

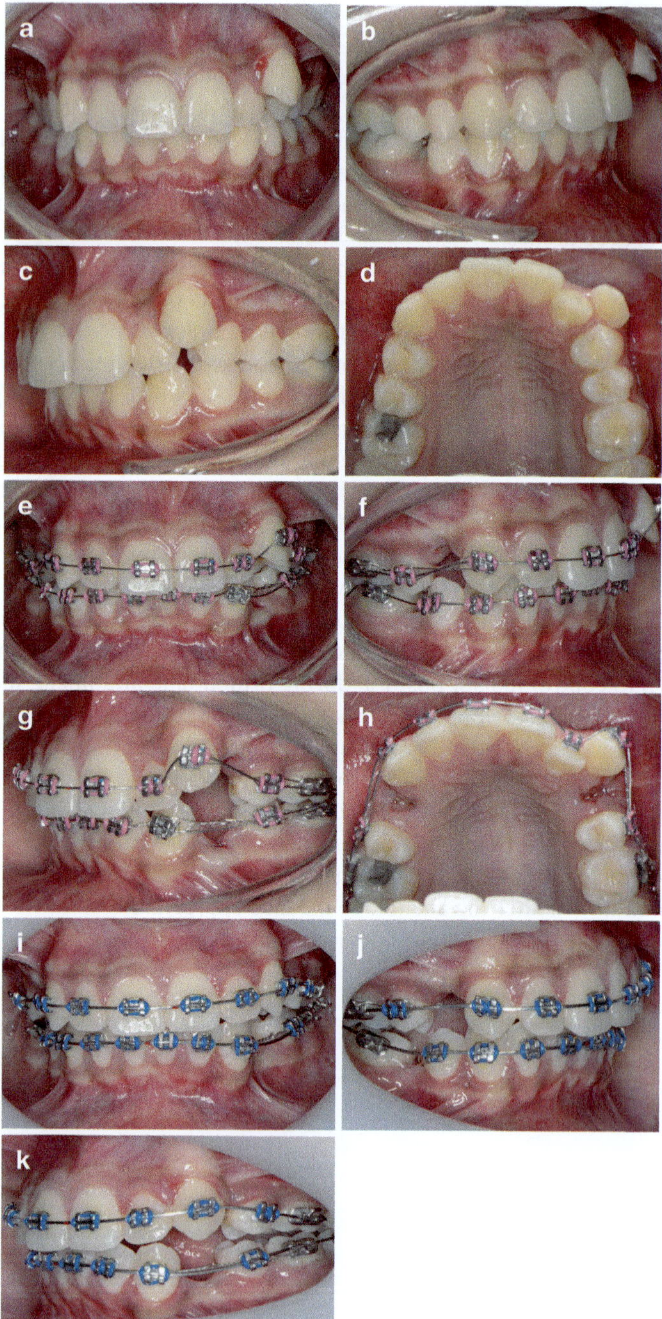

Fig. 4.11 (**a–k**) A crowded Class I malocclusion with buccally displaced maxillary left canine with an associated midline shift to the left side (**a–d**). An initial 0.014-in. NiTi aligning wire was placed with lacebacks from canine to first molar (**e–h**). These assisted in achieving alignment with some distal movement of the canines (**i–k**) prior to definitive space closure in rectangular stainless steel wires

Box 4.3 Self-Ligating Brackets

Self-ligating brackets obviate the need for auxiliaries such as elastomerics or stainless steel ligatures to secure the arch wire in place (see Chap. 1). These brackets incorporate either a slide or clip mechanism offering the potential advantage of secure, constant ligation assuming that the clip or spring does not fatigue or open. This is potentially advantageous in view of the susceptibility of elastomerics, in particular, to degradation and force decay. Claims have been made in relation to an associated acceleration in the rate of orthodontic tooth movement, allied to potential reduction in overall treatment time, primarily ascribed to resistance to sliding associated with the presence of the elastomeric. These claims, however, have largely been refuted in clinical trials, and the primary advantages of self-ligation appear to be a modest saving in relation to chairside time and less requirement for chairside assistance (Fleming and Johal 2010). There is, however, possible merit in the local use of self-ligations to facilitate derotation of severely rotated teeth (Fig. 4.12a–g).

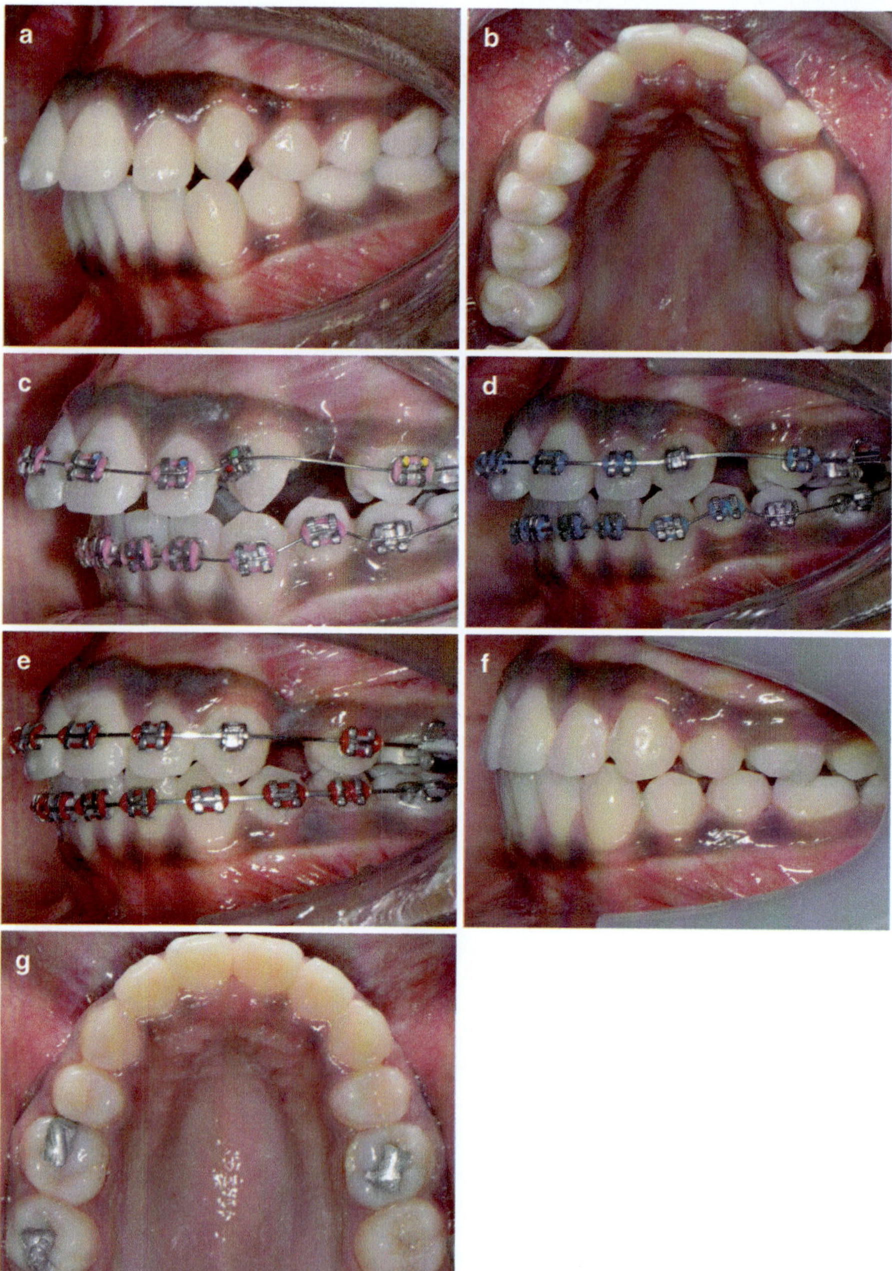

Fig. 4.12 (**a–g**) Local use of a self-ligating bracket on a mesio-palatally rotated maxillary left canine (**a–d**). The secure engagement overcomes the characteristic force degradation of elastomerics and may simplify alignment (**e–g**)

Box 4.4 Duration of Alignment

The initial alignment phase typically spans up to 6 months but may obviously be more prolonged in cases with severe rotations, crowding and tooth displacements (Fig. 4.13a–e). The latter, in particular, may necessitate extractions and sliding mechanics (Chap. 5) with space redistribution prior to inclusion of all anterior teeth within the appliance. Numerous studies investigating the effect of wire and bracket type on the duration of alignment have been undertaken, with less than 8 months usually required prior to engagement of 0.019 × 0.025-in. stainless steel wires in extraction cases (Scott et al. 2008). Little difference has been observed in terms of alignment efficiency with competing wires (Pandis et al. 2009) or bracket designs (Scott et al. 2008). Notwithstanding this, NiTi alloys tend to be preferred to stainless steel alternatives (including multistrand and multiloop designs, which incorporate increased wire length to enhance flexibility) in view of simplicity and resistance to permanent deformation.

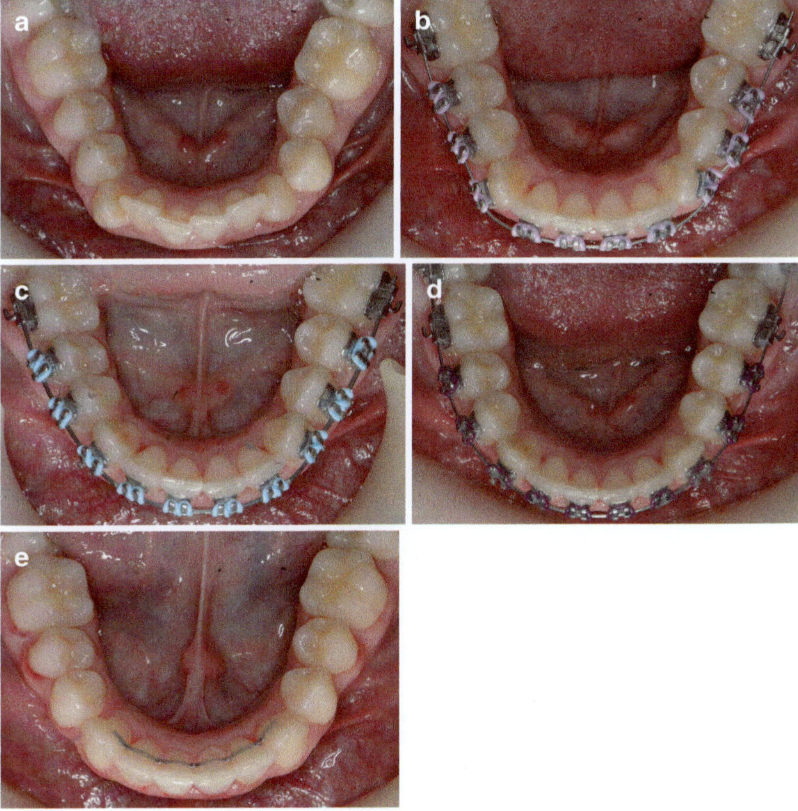

Fig. 4.13 (**a**–**e**) A crowded lower arch (**a**). A decision was made to treat this without extraction allowing advancement of the mandibular incisors. The initial aligning wires were not cinched to allow for arch lengthening. The attachments on the rotated LL3 and LL5 were not fully ligated in 0.014-in. NiTi (**b**); this wire was therefore retied before progressing to rectangular NiTi with complete wire engagement (**c**). The mandibular second molars were subsequently bonded (**d**), and ultimately complete alignment is achieved (**e**)

References

Fleming PS, Johal A. Self-ligating brackets in orthodontics: a systematic review. Angle Orthod. 2010;80(3):575–84.

Irvine R, Power S, McDonald F. The effectiveness of laceback ligatures: a randomized controlled clinical trial. J Orthod. 2004;31(4):303–11.

Kusy RP. A review of contemporary archwires: their properties and characteristics. Angle Orthod. 1997;67(3):197–207.

O'Brien K, Lewis D, Shaw W, Combe E. A clinical trial of aligning archwires. Eur J Orthod. 1990;12(4):380–4.

Pandis N, Polychronopoulou A, Eliades T. Alleviation of mandibular anterior crowding with copper-nickel-titanium vs nickel-titanium wires: a double-blind randomized control trial. Am J Orthod Dentofac Orthop. 2009;136(2):152–e1.

Scott P, DiBiase AT, Sherriff M, Cobourne MT. Alignment efficiency of Damon3 self-ligating and conventional orthodontic bracket systems: a randomized clinical trial. Am J Orthod Dentofac Orthop. 2008;134(4):470–e1.

Space Redistribution 5

Space redistribution is usually undertaken following the initial alignment phase of treatment in the presence of significant crowding and displacements. A dedicated space redistribution or sliding mechanics phase is not usually required in non-extraction cases and is usually reserved for cases with significantly displaced teeth with lack of local, usable space to permit alignment. Teeth are said to require a force, time and space in order to align; lack of usable space may impede tooth movement or lead to inadvertent arch lengthening or loss of arch form during alignment.

In reality, the rationale for extractions or other modes of space creation is usually to address crowding (tooth size-arch length deficiency) with no or minimal increase in arch length. Accordingly, limited or no advancement of the incisors may be desirable. If incisor proclination arises during alignment, the incisors may be retracted later in treatment. This cycle of advancement and retraction has been termed 'round tripping' and may risk slightly greater increments of root resorption allied to possible periodontal attachment loss if excessive proclination of the incisors occurs in susceptible patients.

Space redistribution is usually carried out during sliding or 'push-pull' mechanics, implying that teeth are sliding along a base archwire. It is important that tooth movements are controlled during this treatment phase with light forces in order to limit deleterious effects of active mechanics. Moreover, use of active mechanics risks inducing local rotations; as such, careful ligation remains important during this treatment phase.

P. Fleming, J. Seehra, *Fixed Orthodontic Appliances*, BDJ Clinician's Guides,
https://doi.org/10.1007/978-3-030-12165-5_5

Box 5.1 Rationale for Use of Round Stainless Steel in Sliding Mechanics

Two wire properties are particularly critical in this treatment phase: low resistance to sliding and sufficient rigidity to allow maintenance of arch form. Round stainless steel presents low resistance to sliding in view of the smooth surface configuration with relatively low preponderance of asperities (microscopic peaks) which might impede free sliding (Rossouw 2003). Stainless steel wires are also relatively stiff, therefore resisting arch form changes that might otherwise accompany use of active mechanics such as coil springs and elastomeric chains.

Higher stiffness (lower elastic modulus) would be offered by larger dimension, rectangular steel wires; however, the potential benefit of this should be balanced against the higher resistance to sliding associated with larger wires and the additional time required during the alignment phase to align the slots sufficiently to permit passive engagement of a rectangular steel wire. Notwithstanding this, higher tensile strength round stainless steel wires (e.g. Wilcocks ™ stainless steel; Fig. 5.1) can be considered if greater stiffness and strength is desired during this treatment phase.

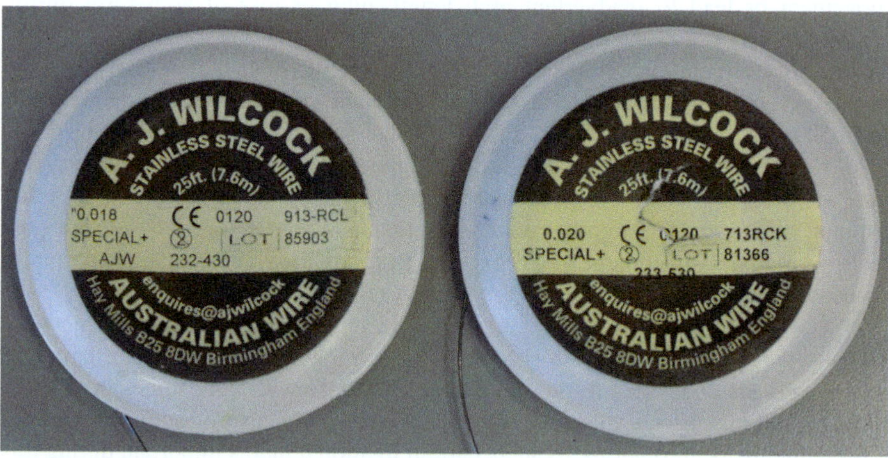

Fig. 5.1 High tensile strength stainless steel wires. These provide additional strength and resilience and were initially used in the Begg appliance as this relied upon use of inter-arch elastics with these resilient wires capable of resisting the elastic force

Box 5.2 Active Mechanics on Nickel-Titanium Wires

Active mechanics are often reserved until placement of more rigid wires to mitigate against adverse arch form changes allied to loss of control of alignment locally due to active force application. For this reason, passive mechanics (e.g. lacebacks) only are used on initial alignment NiTi wires. Notwithstanding this, use of active mechanics can be undertaken earlier with an appreciation that local changes are likely, that light forces are imperative and that over-activation is best avoided. In particular, this approach has been facilitated by metallurgic advancements allied to changes in bracket design. Specifically, self-ligating offers relatively robust ligation potentially limiting the risk of rotations locally, although conventional brackets can also be used on teeth neighbouring active mechanics with judicious ligation. Furthermore, improvement in the strength and superelastic properties of NiTi may assist in resisting the effect of active mechanics in relation to arch form changes (Fig. 5.2a–d).

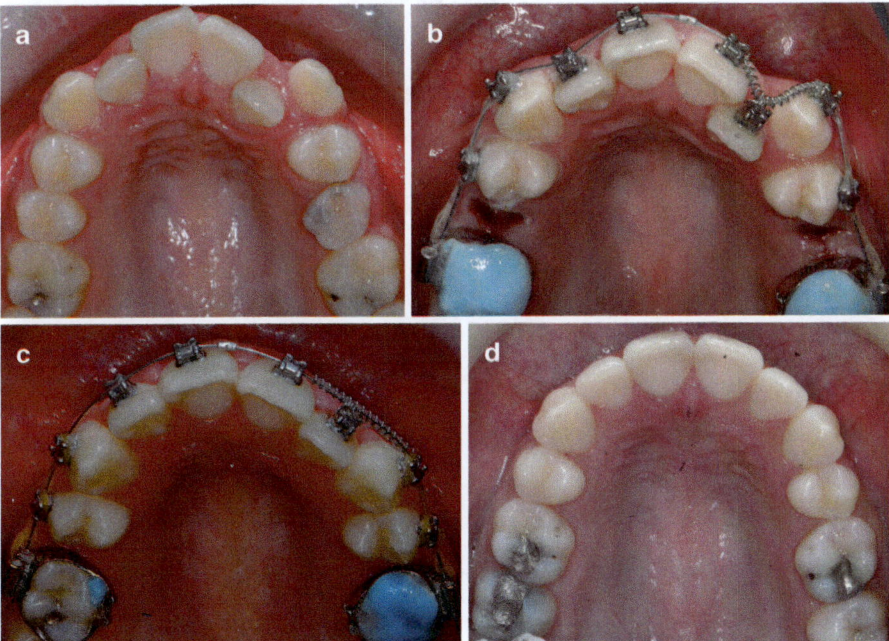

Fig. 5.2 (**a**–**d**) Maxillary arch crowding treated with loss of two premolar units. The anchorage demand in the upper arch was relatively low. Self-ligating brackets were used engaging a 0.013-in. NiTi wire from the outset with active coil spring in the UL2 region. The wire was deflected towards the UL2 attachment using a long ligature thread through the lumen on the attachment. The occlusion was disengaged with glass ionomer cement on the maxillary molars (**b**). Placement of cement on the maxillary rather than mandibular molars is preferable as the cement is easier to remove. Over a 10-week period, the upper left lateral incisor improved in position with distal movement of the canines encouraged with supplementary use of light elastomeric chain (**c**). Ultimately, upper arch alignment was achieved with further labial root torque expression on UL2 (**d**). The secure ligation offered by the self-ligating brackets was exploited here to minimise rotations local to the active mechanics. Moreover, the efficient progress was facilitated by the low anchorage demand; as such, a combination of distal movement of the canines and molar mesial movement contributed to space closure in the premolar region

Box 5.3 Use of Piggyback Wires

Piggyback wires offer the potential to combine wires of similar or, more commonly, markedly different physical properties. In relation to space redistribution and alignment, piggybacks typically involve use of flexible round NiTi wires in combination with more rigid base arch wires permitting alignment of displaced teeth limiting the effect of reactive forces in terms of horizontal and vertical anchorage (Figs. 5.3a–u and 5.9a–i).

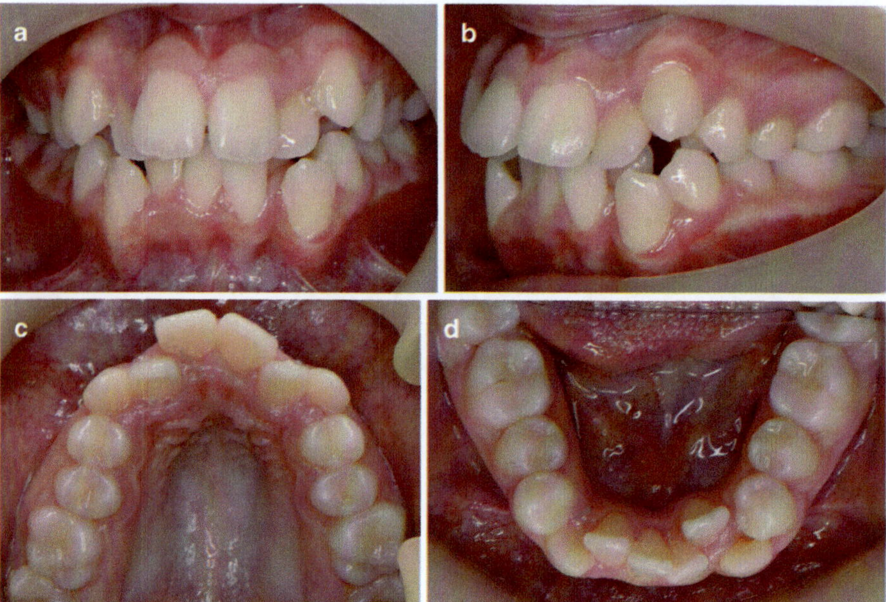

Fig. 5.3 (**a–u**) A Class I malocclusion with severe upper and lower arch crowding treated with loss of four premolar units. Although the maxillary arch was crowded, it was felt that there was sufficient space to align the upper arch without recourse to sliding mechanics. As such, initial alignment was undertaken with NiTi wires engaging all of the teeth from first molar to first molar from the outset before progressing into rectangular wires to permit torque expression on the lateral incisors, in particular (**g, I, o, q**). In the lower arch, there was a lack of space to permit alignment of the left lateral incisor (**b, d**). This tooth was therefore omitted from the appliance initially with engagement of 0.014-in. NiTi and lacebacks in the initial phase. Sliding mechanics was undertaken to redistribute space in the region of the lateral incisor with open coil spring on a 0.018-in. stainless steel base wire. Once sufficient space had been created, an attachment was placed on the LL2, and a piggyback wire is placed. The NiTi coil spring was left in situ passively to prevent space loss during labial movement of the lateral incisor (**e–h**). The piggyback was placed above the steel base wire engaging two teeth on each side of the target tooth with sufficient room distal to the wire to allow free sliding as the incisor aligned. Over a 6-week period, the lateral incisor moved labially with the piggyback sliding distally as the shape memory effect was exerted (**i–k**). Thereafter, a flexible NiTi wire was placed to allow for further alignment (**m, n**) before progression into rectangular wires in the lower arch to permit local torque expression (**p, r**). The lower left lateral incisor was aligned (**s**) and fixed retention utilised to mitigate against maturational change and relapse in view of the extent of the initial irregularity (**t, u**)

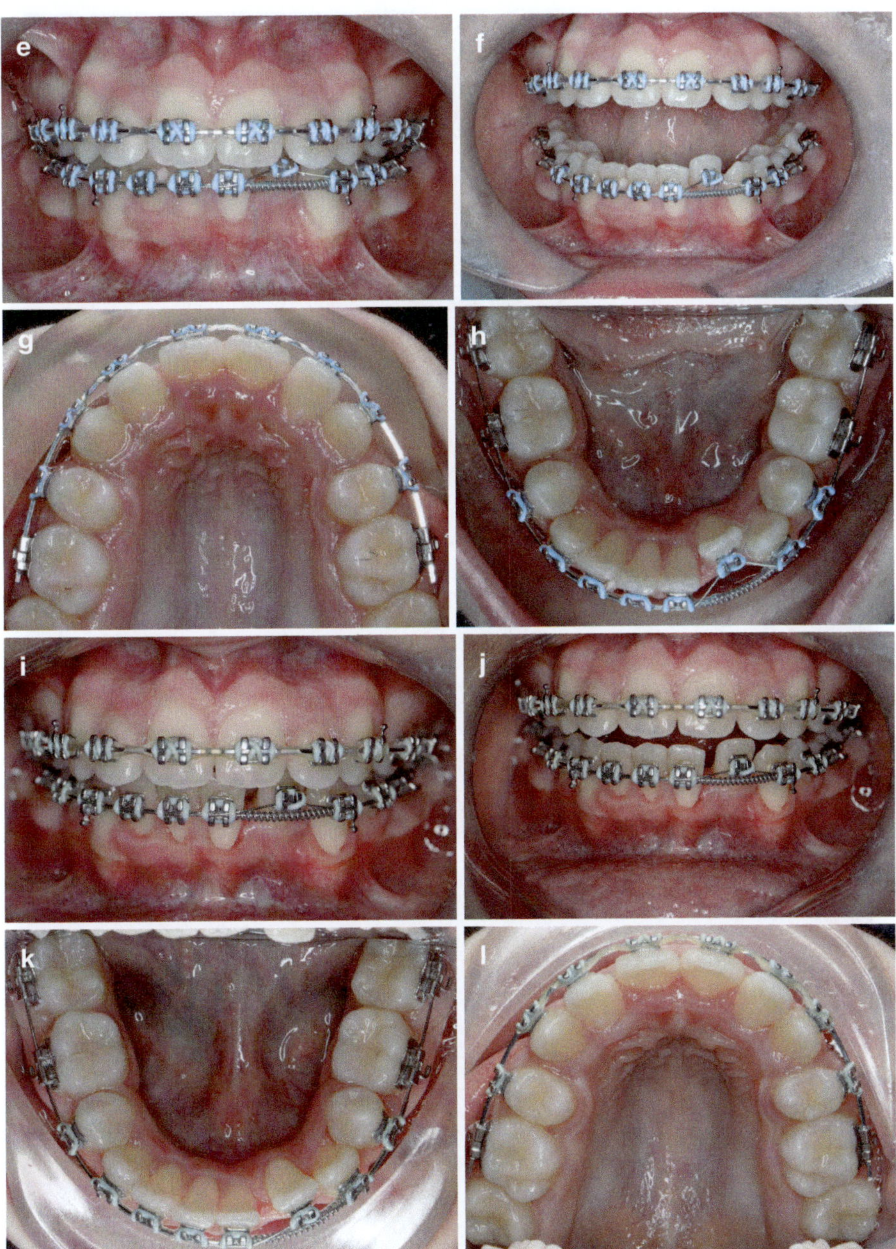

Fig. 5.3 (continued)

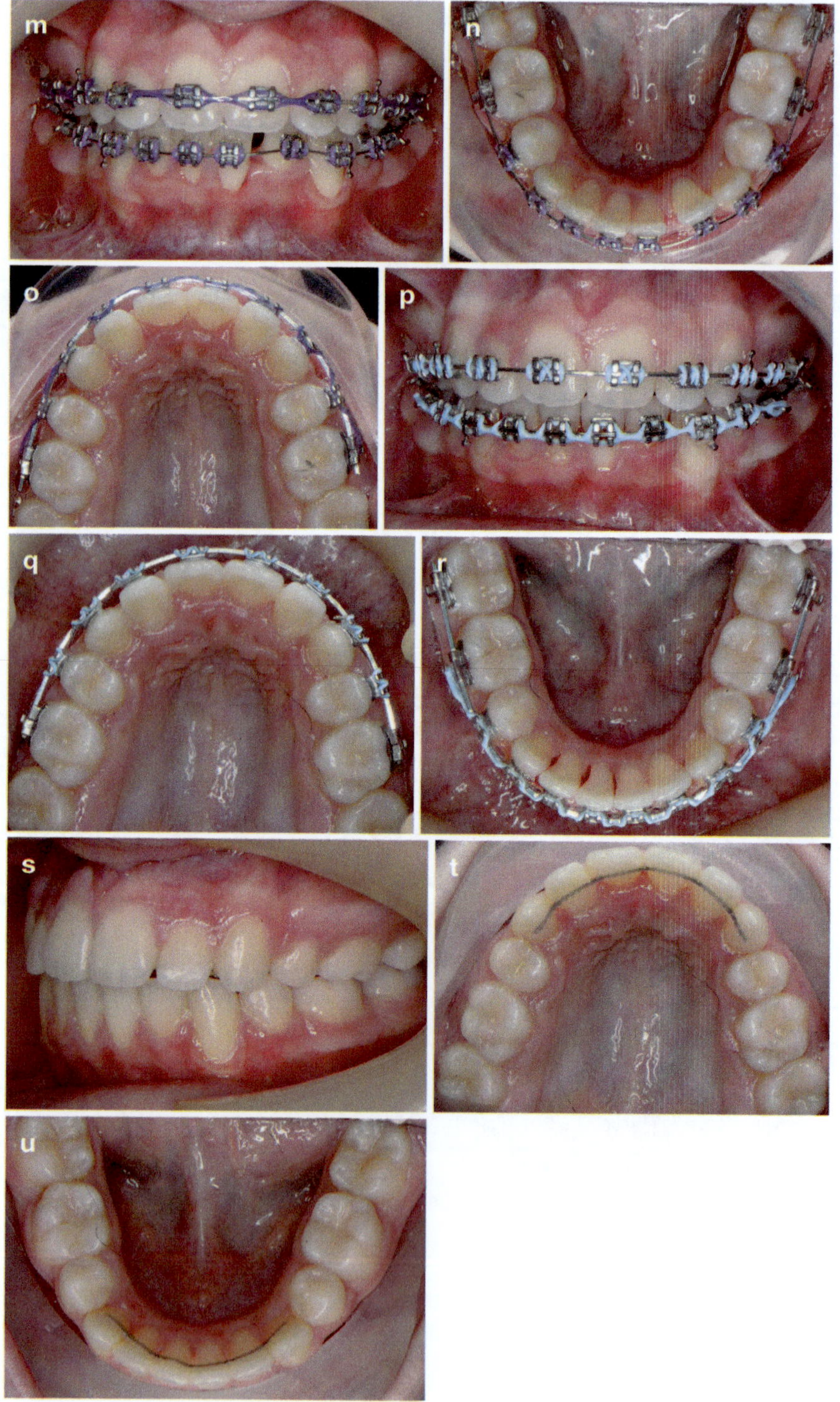

Fig. 5.3 (continued)

Box 5.4 Individual Retraction of Canines

Individual retraction of canines may be undertaken either to localise space for alignment of crowded incisors or potentially to limit anchorage demands. Distal movement of the canines can be performed on a base round stainless steel wire (0.018- or 0.020-in.; Box 5.1). Retraction can be undertaken using elastomeric chain, NiTi coils or sectional springs. In terms of force level, there is little agreement as to the ideal force magnitude required for tooth movement (Ren et al. 2003). However, during space closure there appears to be no increase in rate of tooth movement with force levels above 150 g, although a 150 g force produced more efficient tooth movement than 100 g (Samuels et al. 1998).

Individual retraction of canines may limit the risk of anchorage loss on posterior molar anchor units prior to en masse space closure. Specifically, by retracting the canine into a Class I position, the resultant occlusal interlock may allow preservation of the canine relationship, while space mesial to this tooth is subsequently closed. Evidence in relation to the efficacy of this approach is not compelling, however (Xu et al. 2010). The potential biomechanical advantage should also be weighed against the increased treatment duration required to retract teeth individually prior to complete space closure (Fig. 5.4a–f).

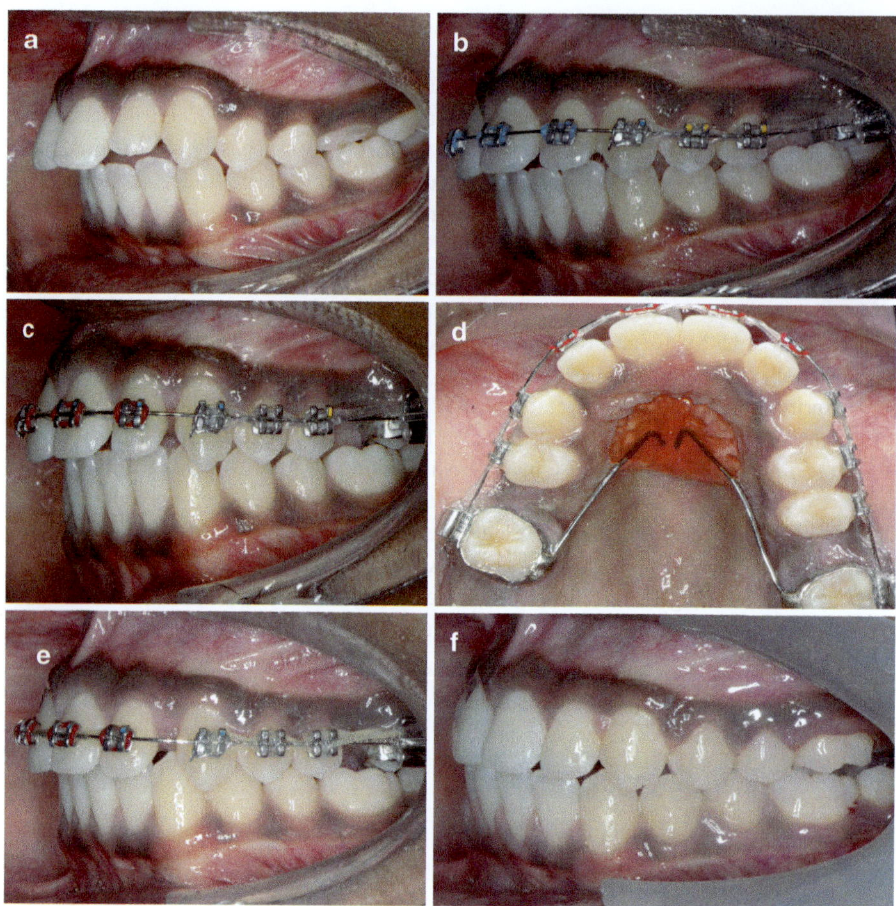

Fig. 5.4 (**a**–**f**) A Class II division 1 incisor relationship with an overjet of 8 mm, reduced overbite and unit II molar relationship on the left side (**a**). The hypoplastic UL6 had a poor long-term prognosis and was therefore extracted in order to facilitate Class II correction and reduction in overjet. The canine relationship was full unit Class II implying a significant anchorage demand to fully reduce the overjet. A Nance palatal arch (**d**) was therefore placed to supplement posterior anchorage. The Nance is believed to provide some degree of anchorage support but does not afford absolute anchorage. As such, sequential retraction of the canine into a Class I relationship was undertaken (**b**–**e**) with elastomeric chain from canine to first molar. Anterior spacing was also consolidated during this phase localising space mesial to the canine. Distal movement was relatively straightforward in this instance as the overbite was reduced; in the presence of increased overbite, distal canine movement can be impeded by interference with the opposing mandibular canine bracket risking anchorage loss and attrition. Overbite reduction or some form of disclusion may therefore be required to allow efficient and effective retraction. Note that steel ligatures are placed on the canines during retraction to mitigate against mesio-buccal rotation during distal movement. Once a Class I relationship had been obtained (**e**), the Nance was discarded and final space closure undertaken permitting full overjet reduction (**f**)

Box 5.5 Cinching of Distal Ends

Cinching of distal ends of round stainless steel wires is typically undertaken during sliding mechanics. Careful cinching reduces the potential for increase in arch length as this is rarely desirable in extraction cases. Space can therefore be redistributed availing of extraction space to allow for alignment of severely displaced teeth. Tight cinching can be undertaken where no increase in arch length is permissible (Fig. 5.5a–c), whereas if minor increases are desirable, the wire can be cinched 1–2 mm distal to the terminal molar tube. It should be pointed out that cinching of terminal ends of NiTi wires is likely not indicated in non-extraction cases where relief of crowding is planned by increase in arch length (often due to incisor proclination and/or transverse expansion).

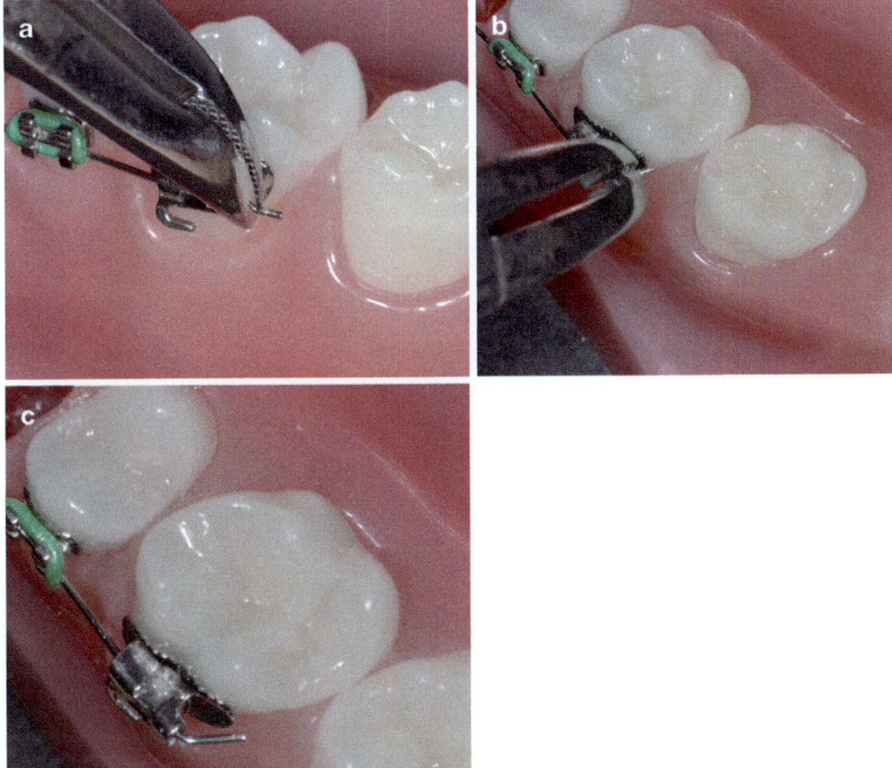

Fig. 5.5 (**a**–**c**) A Weingart pliers may be used to cinch a stainless steel wire (**a**). It is important that the instrument does not lever off the attachment and that bends are made perpendicular to the attachment (horizontally or vertically) to reduce the risk of detachment (**b**, **c**)

5.1 Sliding Mechanics: Practical Steps

Open coil springs can be used to redistribute space local to displaced teeth, often lateral incisors or canines. NiTi coil spring has greater flexibility than stainless steel and may therefore be used with higher degrees of activation using lengths of up to twice the width of the inter-bracket space. With stainless steel push coil, additional coil spring of approx. 1 bracket width can be included (Fig. 5.6a, b). The coil spring is placed on either side using a wire tucker to engage the second attachment (Fig. 5.6c). Stainless steel ligatures are used on the teeth neighbouring the active spring to mitigate against local rotations (Fig. 5.6c). The terminal wire end has been cinched in an effort to fix the arch length permitting distal movement of the canine into the premolar extraction site without inducing advancement of the maxillary incisors (Fig. 5.6d). Reactivation of coil spring can be undertaken in a simple manner using stainless steel (crimpable) stops crimped into position using Weingart's pliers without the requirement to remove the base archwire (Fig. 5.6e–h). Flowable composite can be used as an alternative, although this is more prone to loss.

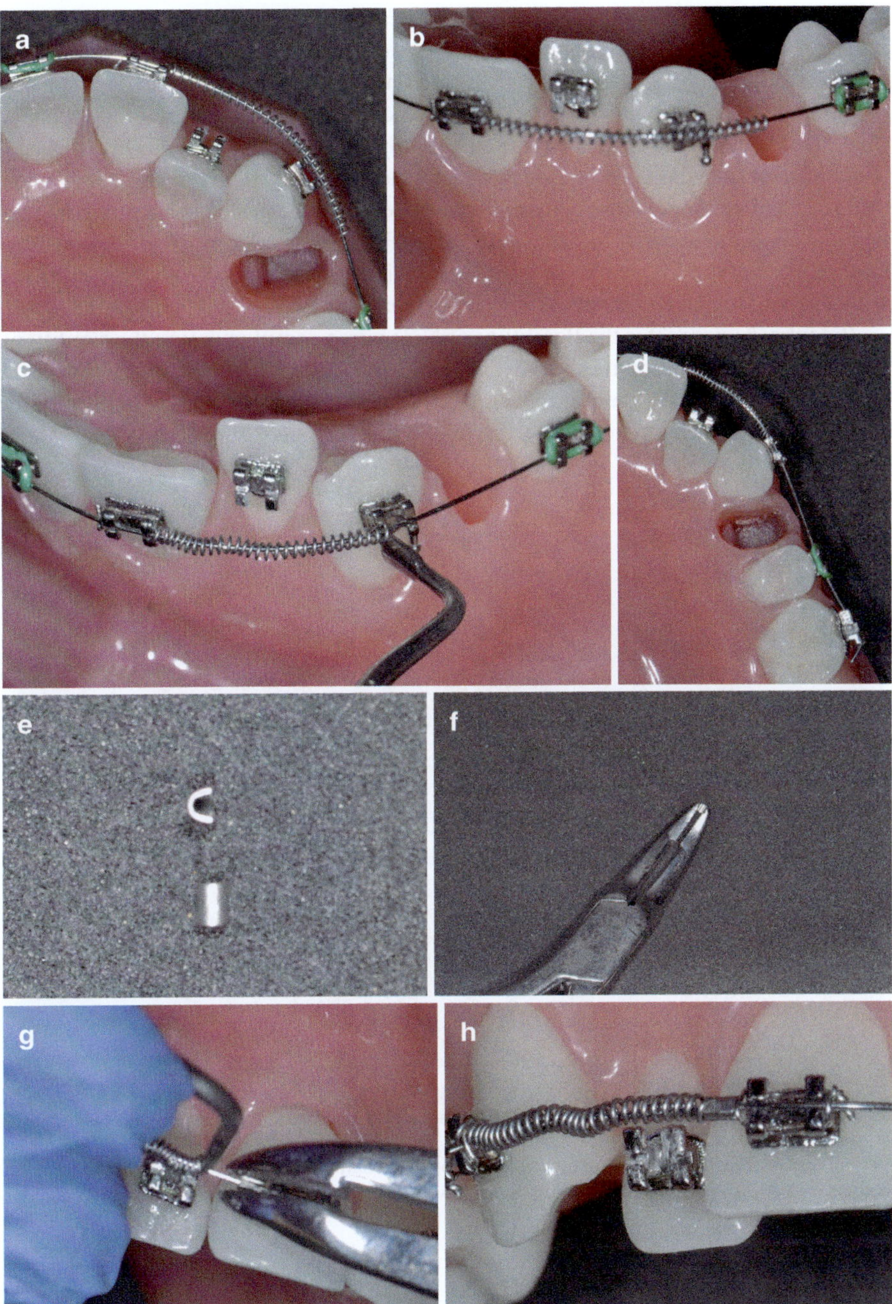

Fig. 5.6 (**a-h**) Placement (**a-d**) and reactivation (**e-h**) of NiTi open coil-spring for space redistribution

Elastomeric chain to retract individual teeth can be applied using mosquito forceps. In the example shown, the chain is being used to aid retraction of the canine into the premolar site (Fig. 5.7). The chain can be held on the end link with the tip of the instrument not obscuring the lumen. This permits placement of the chain in a fluid manner (Fig. 5.7a) with the mosquito being used to apply the first and last links (Fig. 5.7a–d), while intermediate links can be guided into position manually with fingers. Elastomeric chain to facilitate initial alignment of displaced teeth can be placed in a similar manner with the elastomeric being formed into a lasso (Fig. 5.8a–e). Alternatives include elastomeric thread in conjunction with either self-ligating brackets or other attachments with a central lumen to simplify elastomeric engagement.

Piggyback wires offer the flexibility of NiTi wires complementing the rigidity of base stainless steel archwires which are used for space redistribution during sliding mechanics (Box 5.3). The piggyback can be engaged on the target tooth initially before gently ligating to adjacent teeth above the base steel wire (Fig. 5.9a–i).

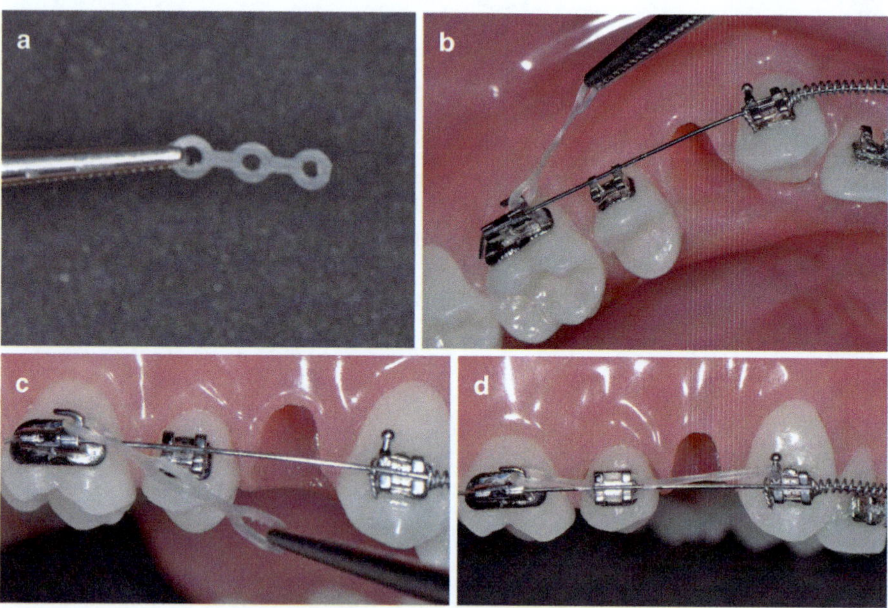

Fig. 5.7 (**a-d**) Placement of open (spaced) elastomeric chain to retract the maxillary canine. This may be undertaken in isolation or in conjunction with coil-spring locally during push-pull (sliding) mechanics

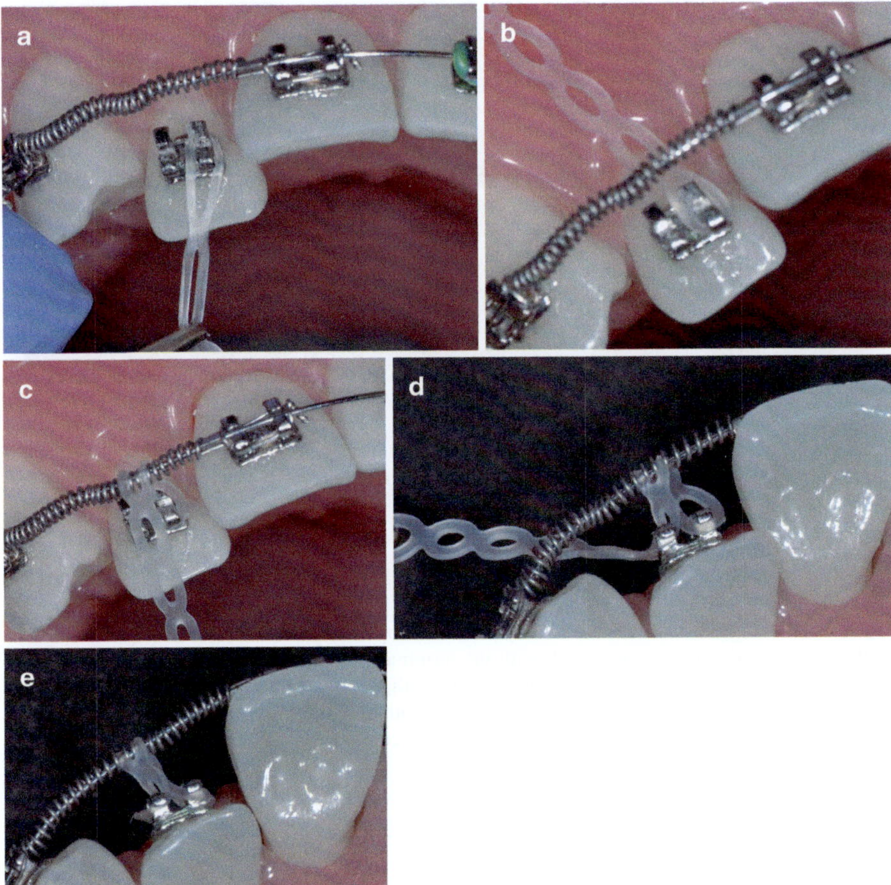

Fig. 5.8 (**a**-**e**) Elastomeric chain placed as a lasso to facilitate labial movement of the displaced lateral incisor

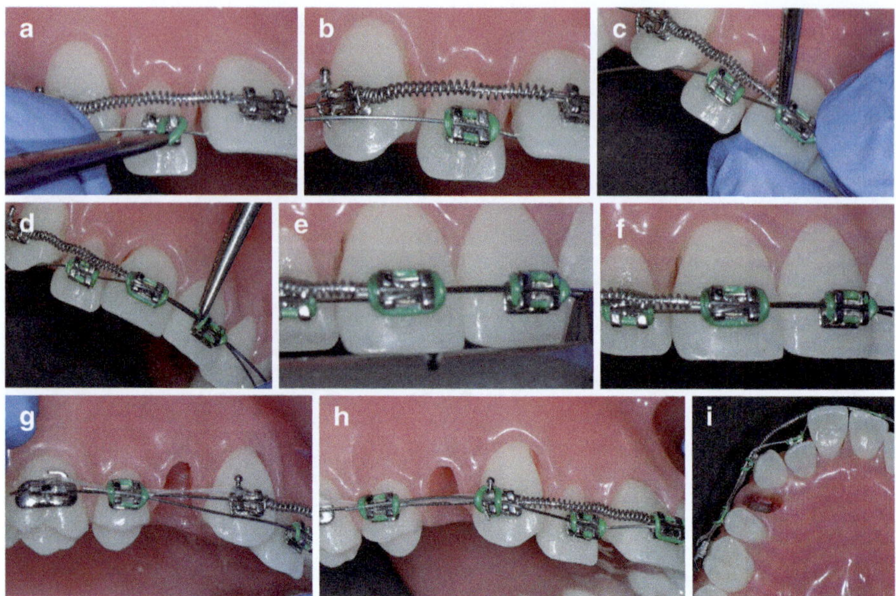

Fig. 5.9 (**a**–**i**) Piggyback wires are usually placed on top of the base wire with engagement of two teeth on either side of the target tooth with the terminal ends of the wire ending just distal to an attachment to permit sliding as the displaced tooth is aligned (**e**). The inclusion of two attachments reduces the risk of breakages as ligation to a single tooth only risks disengagement of the wire. On the contrary, inclusion of more than two teeth may increase resistance to sliding impairing tooth movement (**a**–**i**)

References

Ren Y, Maltha JC, Kuijpers-Jagtman AM. Optimum force magnitude for orthodontic tooth movement: a systematic literature review. Angle Orthod. 2003;73(1):86–92.

Rossouw PE. Friction: an overview. Semin Orthod. 2003;9(4):218–22.

Samuels RH, Rudge SJ, Mair LH. A clinical study of space closure with nickel-titanium closed coil springs and an elastic module. Am J Orthod Dentofac Orthop. 1998;114(1):73–9.

Xu TM, Zhang X, Oh HS, Boyd RL, Korn EL, Baumrind S. Randomized clinical trial comparing control of maxillary anchorage with 2 retraction techniques. Am J Orthod Dentofac Orthop. 2010;138(5):544–e1.

Overbite

6

Overbite reduction is a key element of orthodontic treatment, particularly in Class II division 2 malocclusion. Traditionally, during isolated fixed appliance therapy, overbite reduction follows the alignment phase and precedes overjet reduction and space closure. This involves levelling of the curve of Spee in the lower arch with relative extrusion of the posterior teeth and is reliant on engagement of stiff stainless steel lower arch wires of large dimension (e.g. 0.019 × 0.25-in.) often with exaggerated reversed curves to promote further extrusion (Chap. 9). Increasingly, however, earlier overbite reduction can be considered using a range of adjuncts and techniques during the initial alignment phase.

6.1 Mechanisms of Overbite Reduction

Overbite reduction can be affected by anterior intrusion, posterior extrusion, proclination of the anteriors or a combination of these movements (Naini et al. 2006). As with any other occlusal feature, the aetiology of deep overbite should be established in order to tailor treatment accordingly. This requires a full clinical assessment, often supplemented with cephalometric analysis, in order to assess key features such as lower anterior facial height, Frankfurt-mandibular planes angle, incisal display at rest (Box 6.1) and on smiling and occlusal curves.

Posterior extrusion (or relative extrusion) involves arch levelling with flattening of increased occlusal curves, particularly in the lower arch. This leads to an increase in lower anterior facial height and may be accompanied by proclination of the lower anteriors as there is a space requirement to level the contact points. The tendency to procline can, however, be limited with space creation (Box 6.2) and judicious wire bending, specifically addition of labial root torque to the lower incisors.

P. Fleming, J. Seehra, *Fixed Orthodontic Appliances*, BDJ Clinician's Guides,
https://doi.org/10.1007/978-3-030-12165-5_6

True intrusion of the incisors is typically indicated in instances with relatively normal facial heights where the incisor teeth are relatively extruded. This may manifest as increased incisal display at rest and with gingival exposure on smiling. The capacity to produce true incisor intrusion is limited (Ng et al. 2005). Segmental approaches including Ricketts and Burstone mechanics have been used as a means of producing true intrusion. More recently mini-implants offer the potential to produce isolated intrusion of teeth without producing reciprocal extrusion of posterior teeth and concomitant increase in facial height.

Proclination is an effective means of reducing overbite with each five degrees of proclination leading to overbite decrease of the order of 1 mm (Eberhart et al. 1990). Proclination of the lower anteriors is considered unstable (Mills 1966), although it has been postulated that advancement in lower incisors in Class II division 2 cases may offer better levels of stability (Selwyn-Barnett 1996). This has not been proven; however, there is an undoubted mechanical benefit to allowing proclination and advancement of the lower incisors in these cases.

Box 6.1 Maxillary Incisor Display and Age

A key arbiter of the approach to overbite reduction is the incisal display at rest and on smiling. Approximately, 3–4 mm and 2–3 mm of incisal display at rest in male and female adolescents, respectively, are considered normal. However, changes in lip thickness, tone and length during adulthood lead to a decrease in incisal exposure at rest with da Motta et al. (2010) estimating a decrease of just under 1 mm per decade from 15 to 50 years from 4.5 mm to 1.3 mm in females and 3.3 mm to 0.6 mm in males. In terms of lip mobility and tooth and gingival exposure on smiling, lip length has been shown to reduce by approx. 30% on full smiling exposing up to 2 mm of gingivae (Roe et al. 2012). With more expressive lip behaviour, more gingival display may result, and a decision may therefore be required in relation to whether to plan vertical incisor positioning in relation to the rest or smile position.

Box 6.2 Extractions and Overbite

Mandibular arch extractions and overbite are generally considered antagonistic. As such, lower arch extractions in deep overbite cases, particularly with Class II division 2 type incisor relationships, are typically best avoided. This approach does place an onus on diligent prolonged retention in the lower arch to resist the tendency to post-treatment uprighting of the mandibular incisors, leading to return of lower anterior crowding and consequent increase in the overbite. However, advancement of the lower incisors may also induce subtle soft tissue profile changes, the latter may be of some benefit in this subset of patients as Class II division 2 type malocclusion is often accompanied by a retrusive soft tissue profile. Clearly, however, the relative merits of change in the anteroposterior position of the lower incisors should be evaluated as part of a holistic assessment of facial and occlusal features, as well as the predictability of the desired outcome.

Lower arch extractions tend to complicate effective overbite reduction for the following reasons:

- Reduced tendency to advance and procline mandibular incisors: Extraction decisions are based on an overall evaluation of treatment objectives and space requirements to address these. With limited crowding and retroclined incisors, extractions may create excessive space hindering any planned advancement or proclination of the incisors.
- Less effective arch levelling: Extrusion of the premolars relative to the incisors, in particular, is a key element of arch levelling. Extraction of premolars renders this levelling less effective.
- Extrusion of incisors: Extraction of incisors may be accompanied by their posterior movement and associated extrusion.
- 'Anti-wedge' effect: Posterior extractions are often accompanied by a degree of mesial movement of posterior teeth as a consequence of anchorage loss. By moving the posterior occlusal wedge anteriorly, the overbite tends to increase. As such, posterior extractions, and indeed extractions of terminal molars, are a recognised means of increasing overbite in anterior open bites (Kim 1987; Sarver and Weissman 1995).

Upper arch extractions have a less profound influence on the overbite and may be considered where Class II correction is required, although distal molar movement with a range of adjuncts including a ten Hoeve appliance in conjunction with headgear (Fig. 6.1a–k), use of fixed Class II correctors or temporary anchorage devices may be considered as alternatives.

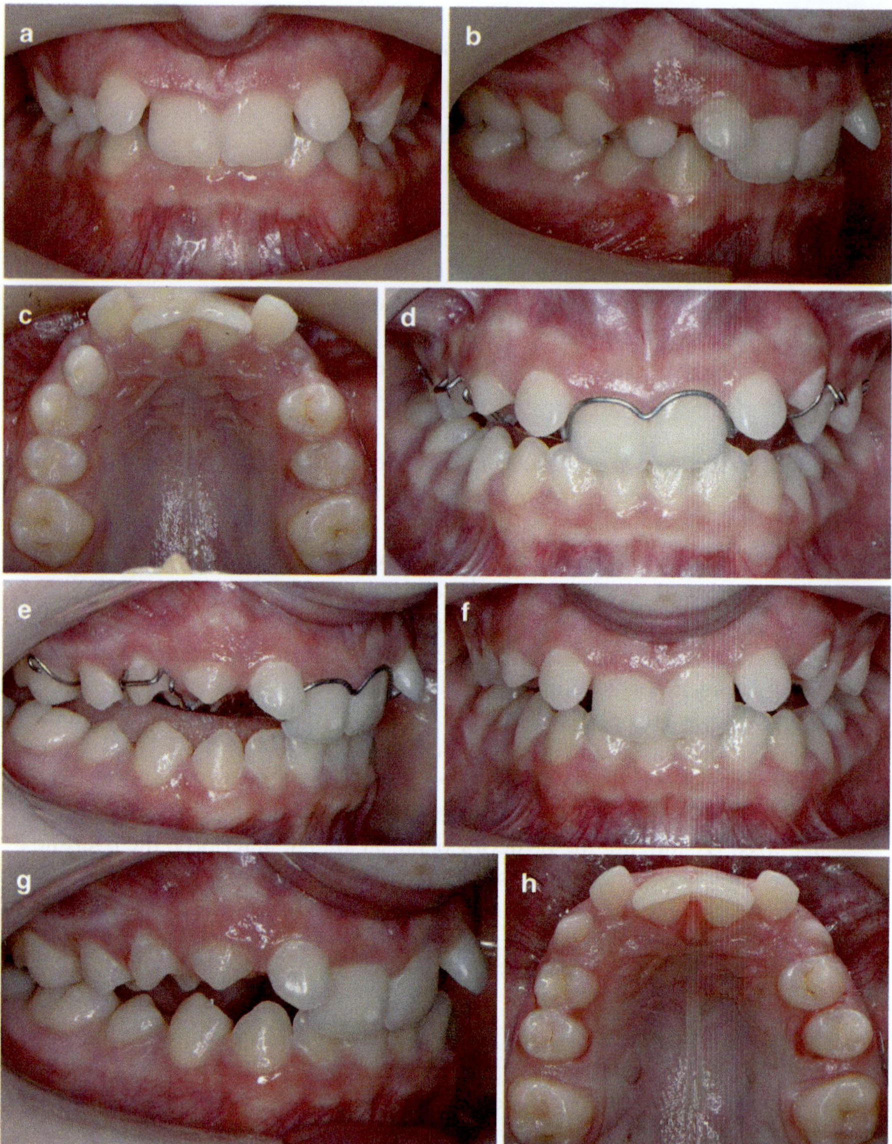

Fig. 6.1 (**a**–**k**) A classic Class II division 2 type malocclusion with increased overbite and proclined maxillary lateral incisors with half unit Class II molar relationship in the mixed dentition (**a**–**c**). A ten Hoeve-type appliance was fitted for full-time wear with a flat anterior bite plane. Retention was provided by anterior clasping with a Southend clasp as well as an Adams' crib on the maxillary first premolars (**d**, **e**). Diligent wear resulted in overbite reduction allied to distal movement of the first permanent molars producing molar correction over a 6-month period (**f**–**h**). A lower fixed appliance was subsequently placed to consolidate arch levelling with maintenance of the upper removable appliance at night before an upper fixed appliance was placed to align the teeth and detail the occlusion (**i**–**k**)

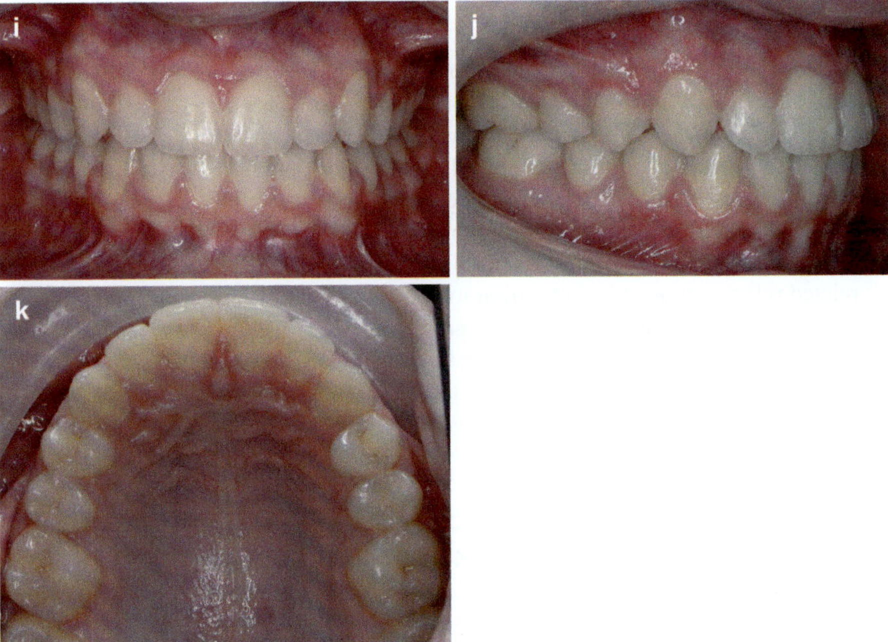

Fig. 6.1 (continued)

Box 6.3 Arch Levelling and Space Requirement

Arch levelling may be considered in the lower arch, in particular, as a means of overbite reduction. In the maxillary arch, an increased curve of Spee can be added if maxillary incisor intrusion and advancement is required, perhaps where the maxillary incisors appear elongated with excessive incisal or gingival display at rest or on smiling. However, levelling of the lower curve of Spee represents a more fundamental method of overbite reduction. This involves extrusion of the lower posterior teeth, including premolars and first molar. It is facilitated by use of stiff base arch wires, incorporating reverse curves, bonding of terminal molars and to an extent by anterior disclusion (although this also produces intrusion of the incisors). Levelling of contact points entails a space requirement, and formal approaches to space planning tend to apportion a space requirement to this procedure (Kirschen et al. 2000). This has been estimated at 1 mm for 3 mm, 1.5 mm for 4 mm and 2 mm for 5 mm of depth reduction.

Box 6.4 Stability of Overbite Reduction

Overbite reduction is not known to be overly stable; however, relapse in overbite is not necessarily independent of sagittal correction and maintenance of lower anterior alignment with increase in overjet and recurrence of lower anterior crowding with lingual displacement of incisors both predisposing to increased overbite. As such, preservation of perfect alignment as well as antero-posterior stability increase the potential for stable overbite correction. Based on a post-retention study a mean of 15 years following retention, Kim and Little (1999) related relapse in overbite correction to upright pretreatment incisors and depth of the initial overbite with vertical growth a potential predictor of stability. However, in a further study in which 23 of the 30 participants remained in some form of retention (Schütz-Fransson et al. 2006), more encouraging results were reported with overbite increasing by just 0.8 mm in an 11-year follow-up.

6.2 Overbite Reduction: Practical Steps

6.2.1 Fixed Anterior Bite Planes

Fixed anterior bite planes may be placed on one or more maxillary incisor creating posterior disclusion (Figs. 6.2a–g and 6.4a–f). These permit a combination of anterior intrusion and posterior extrusion. Bite planes can be made from customised acrylic or metal components as well as dental adhesive materials (including glass ionomer cement and composite resin). Bite planes may be poorly tolerated as they do involve an increase in the vertical dimension and may interfere with chewing in the short term particularly. Notwithstanding this, they are very potent indeed potentially resulting in 'over-intrusion' of teeth locally; as such, incremental reduction of bite planes may sometimes be undertaken to mitigate against this. The authors therefore currently have a preference for dental adhesives especially glass ionomer (Fig. 6.2) in view of ease of manipulation, incremental reduction and refinement. A small residue of adhesive can be left on the palatal surface until the end of treatment (Fig. 6.2e) allowing sufficient inter-occlusal space for placement of an upper bonded retainer at debond (Fig. 6.2g).

6.2.2 Inclusion of Second Molars

Bonding of second molars is considered integral to lower arch levelling. Lower second molars are typically included relatively early in treatment and may be bonded from the outset or slightly later. Inclusion of second molars from the first visit does predispose somewhat to appliance breakages both in relation to the attachment themselves (particularly where the overbite is deep) but also due to disengagement of flexible wires in view of longer spans between molar tubes. As such,

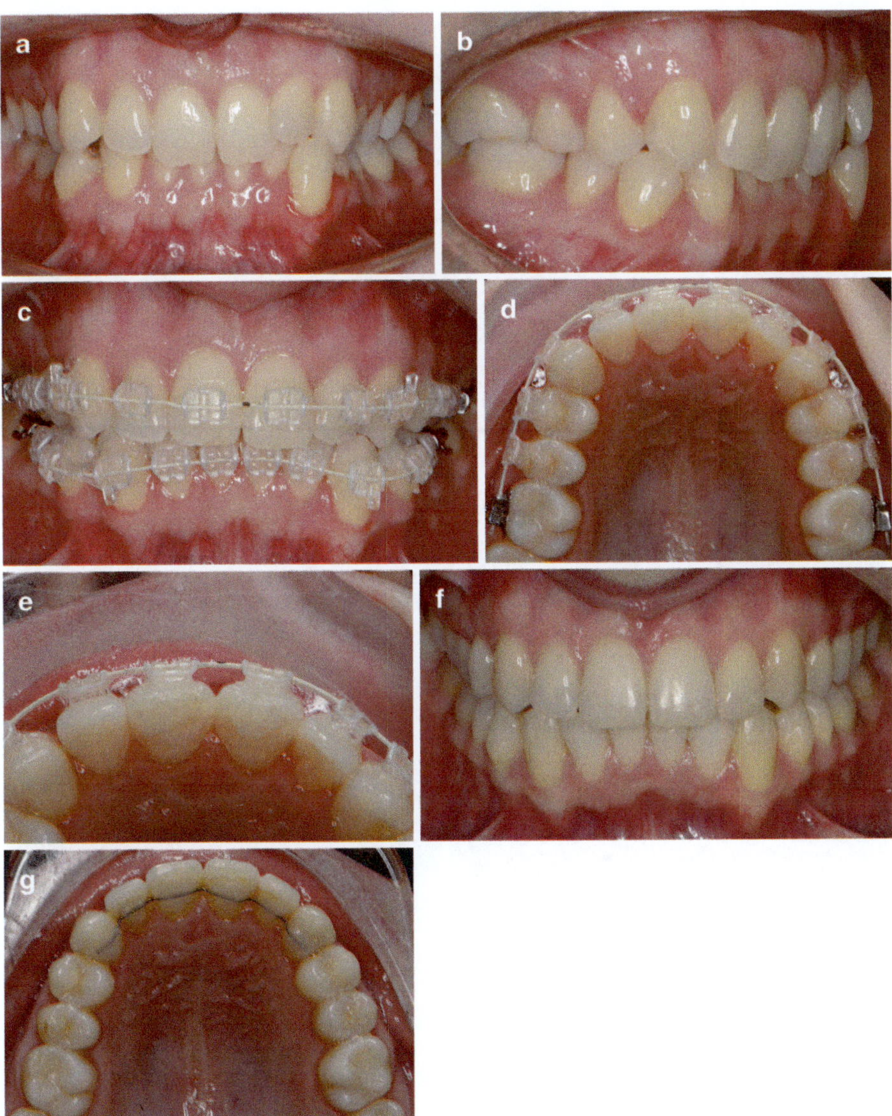

Fig. 6.2 (**a**–**g**) Light-cured glass ionomer is added to the palatal surfaces of the maxillary incisors using a flat plastic instrument. This allows for early reduction in the overbite (**c**) with the thickness reduced over time permitting unimpeded placement of a bonded wire in the space vacated by the cement upon removal

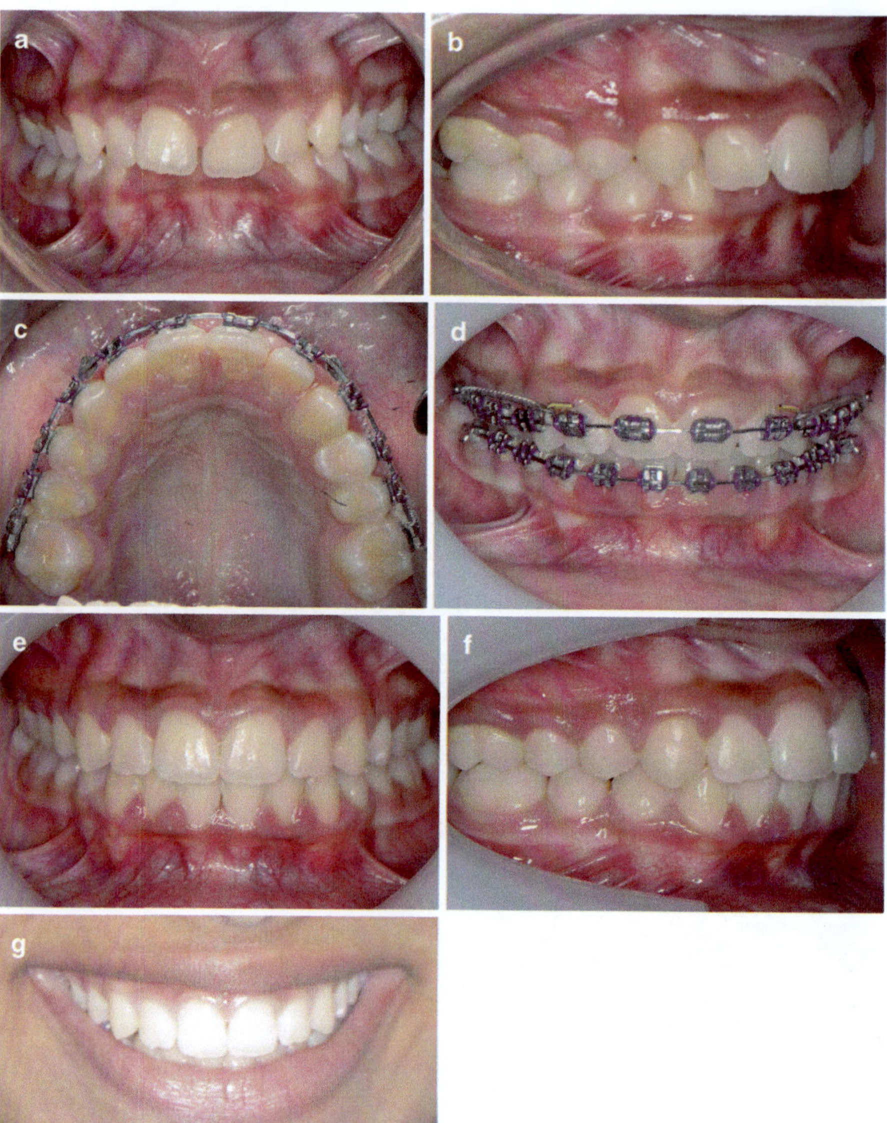

Fig. 6.3 (**a**–**g**) A Class II division 2 type malocclusion with increased overbite and Class I molar relationships (**a**, **b**) was treated with fixed appliances with adjunctive use of a fixed anterior bite plane to allow anterior disclusion and overbite reduction by a combination of anterior intrusion and posterior eruption in a growing patient. Triad gel was placed on both upper central incisors. It is important that these are positioned so as to contact the lower incisal edges in order to facilitate overbite reduction. Moreover, if the mandibular incisors occlude posterior to these, there is a risk of accentuating the overjet and complicating overbite reduction. As such, the bite plane has been positioned mesially on the rotated central incisors (**c**). Fixed bite planes can be particularly potent and my lead to excessive local intrusion (**d**). This was later corrected with local bends (**e**) with the overbite fully reduced producing good smile aesthetics with full tooth display and minimal gingival display on smiling (**g**)

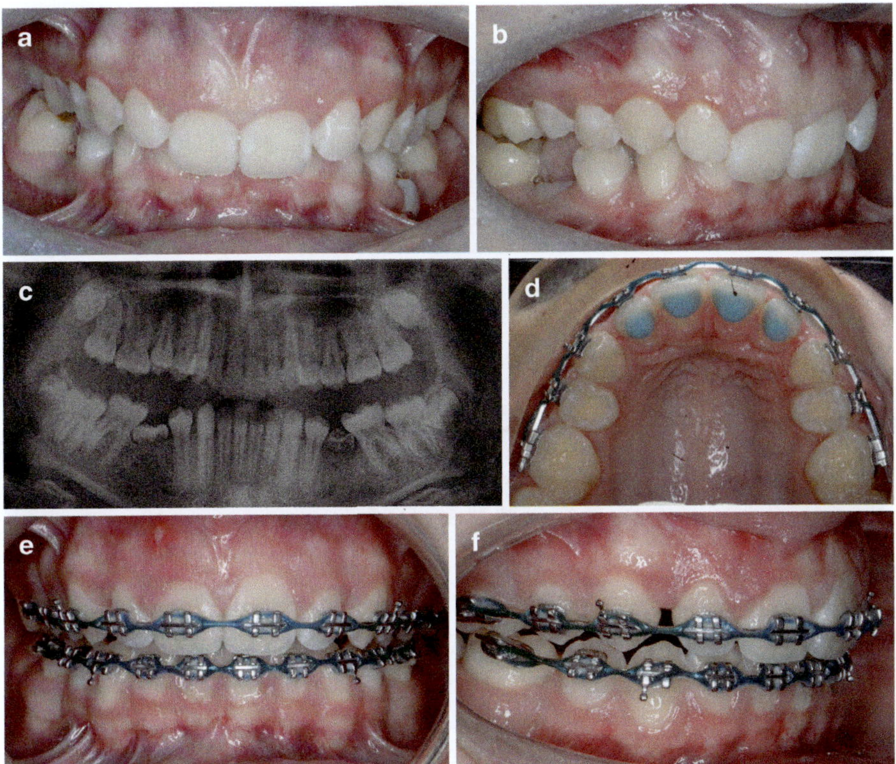

Fig. 6.4 (**a**–**f**) A Class II division 2 type malocclusion with increased overbite with unerupted second molars (**a**–**c**). A decision was made to space close for the missing lower second premolars. This placed a significant premium on overbite reduction as space closure risked accentuating the deep overbite and second molars were not available for bonding. Moreover, treatment duration was likely to be prolonged in view of the significant amount of lower arch space closure required. As such, use of a removable appliance prior to placement of fixed appliances risked leading to excessive treatment time. Glass ionomer cement was placed palatal to all four maxillary incisors (**d**) facilitating overbite reduction and relatively seamless space closure (**e**, **f**)

bonding of second molars may be deferred until larger dimension round (0.018- or 0.020-in.) or rectangular (0.018 × 0.025-in.) NiTi wires are introduced. The effect of second molars on overbite correction is not fully understood but may lead to more effective extrusion of lower first molars and second premolars and may induce angulation changes of the first molars predisposing to overbite reduction. Moreover, allied to the effect on the overbite, bonding of second molars in lower second premolar extraction cases is important in limited unwanted mesial tipping of first molars during space closure.

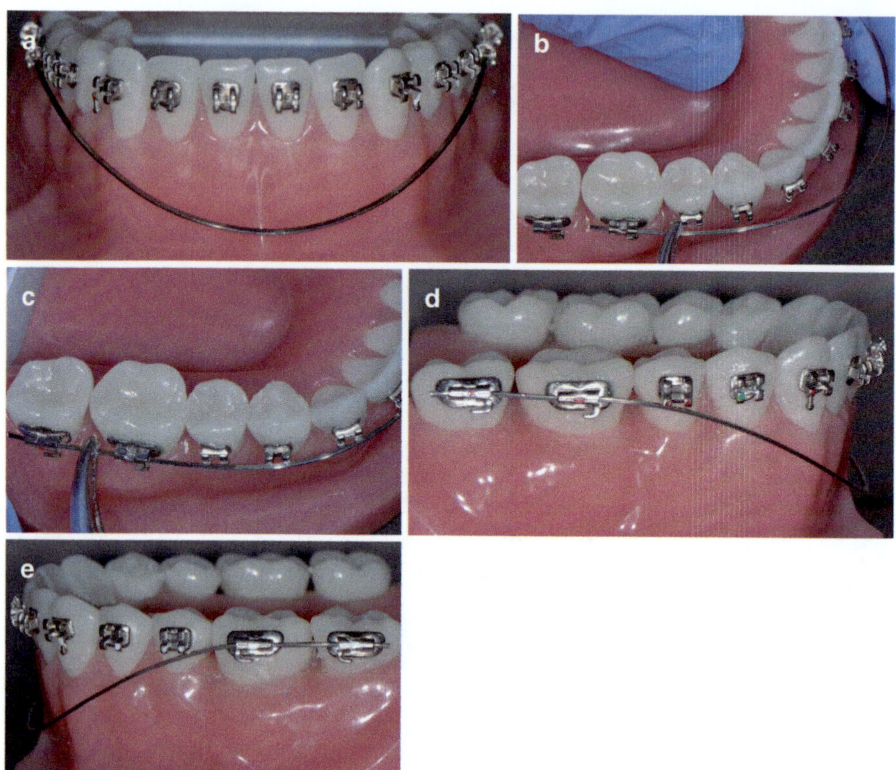

Fig. 6.5 (**a–e**) A 0.019 × 0.025-in. reverse curve NiTi wire. The magnitude of the reverse curve is clear (**a–e**). The latter complicates engagement slightly. The wire can be introduced into the first molar tube using the fingers in the usual way; however, insertion in the second molar tubes requires use of a pliers such as a Weingarts (**b**, **c**) with stabilisation of the wire anteriorly in order to facilitate anterior engagement minimising soft tissue trauma (**b**)

6.2.3 Reverse Curve NiTi (Rocking Chair Wires)

Prefabricated wires with pronounced reverse curves of Spee are an option to facilitate arch levelling (Fig. 6.5a–e). These have the advantages inherent in the flexibility of NiTi permitting full engagement at an earlier stage than stainless steel, therefore achieving arch levelling earlier in treatment. A limitation of these is that they are not 'fail-safe' as the reverse curve is typically excessive. Close supervision and regular recall are therefore advisable.

6.2.4 Rectangular Steel Wire with Reversed Curve of Spee

Rectangular steel (typically 0.019 × 0.025-in.) wires can be formed to produce a reversed curve of Spee encouraging extrusion of the lower buccal segments (Fig. 6.6a–f). These sweeps are introduced manually with care taken to ensure

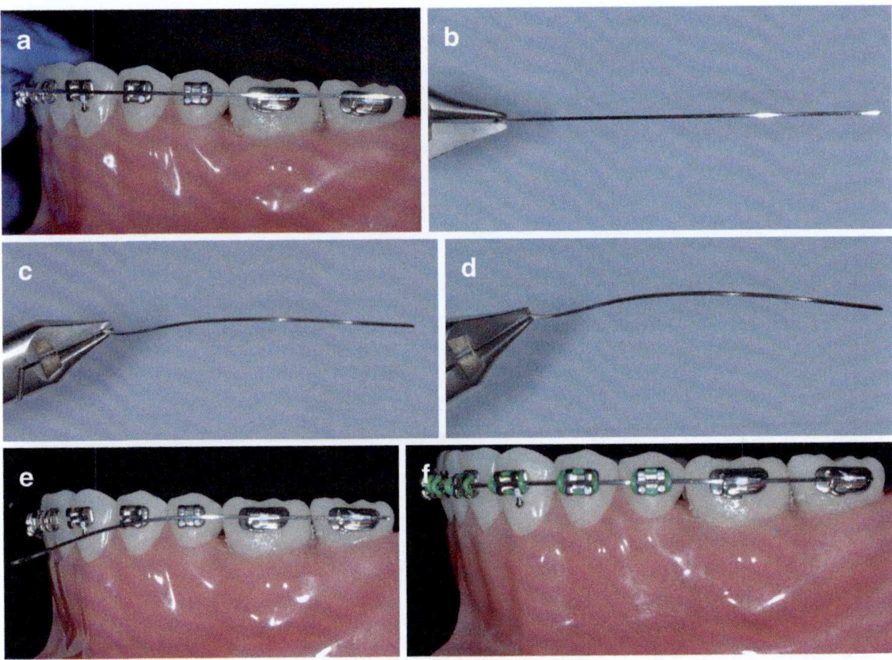

Fig. 6.6 (**a–f**) A 0.019 × 0.025-in. stainless steel wire (**a**, **b**) with reverse curve of Spee of 3–4 mm in depth in the premolar region (**c–e**). The depth of curve can be estimated from the incisal tips to the distal of the occlusal surface of the first molars. The wire is inserted in a similar manner to the reverse curve NiTi with anterior engagement initially to afford sufficient flexibility (**f**)

they are symmetrical and do not disturb the arch form. Compensatory labial root torque adjustment can be added anteriorly in order to counteract the risk of proclination of mandibular incisors in view of the geometric effects of the introduction of the curve allied to the space requirement associated with levelling.

6.2.5 Inter-arch Elastics

Inter-arch elastics tend to have an extrusive effect. Class II elastics run from lower molars to upper anterior teeth and lead to extrusion of the lower molars and maxillary incisors. As the molars are closer to the terminal hinge axis of the mandible, the overall effect is reduction in the overbite. Incisor extrusion can also be limited with introduction of increased curve of Spee in the upper archwire. Elastic configuration can also be varied to encourage further posterior extrusion and arch levelling (Fig. 6.7a, b). Elastics are typically stretched by 2 to 3 times their original length to produce the appropriate force level with near full-time wear encouraged to produce significant change. Nights only wear, however, can be recommended to maintain previous changes.

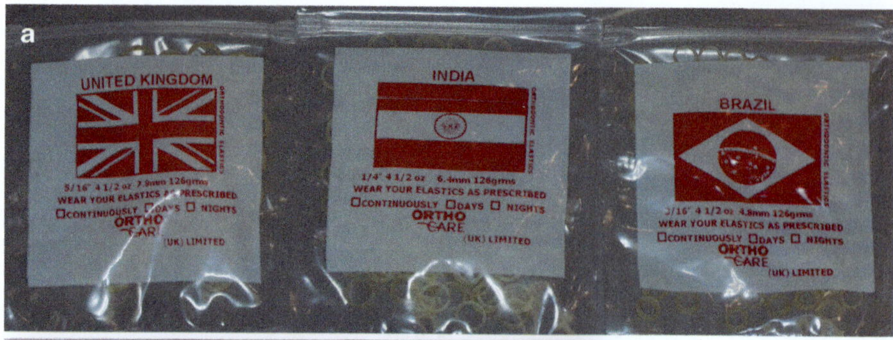

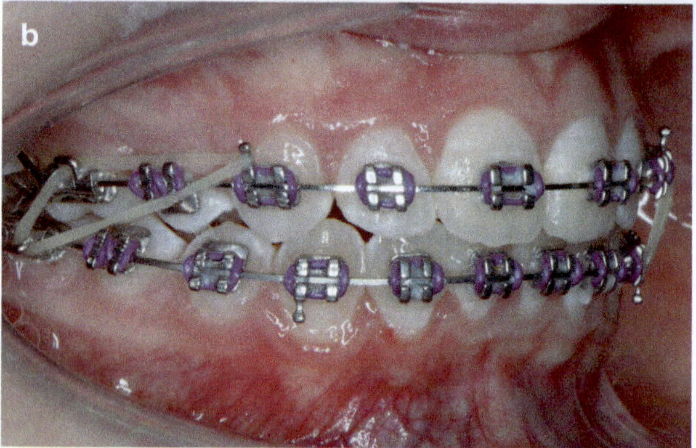

Fig. 6.7 (**a**, **b**) Intra-oral elastics of various lengths. In this instance, stretching of elastics up to three times their original length will produce 126 g of force. Inter-arch elastics tend to have an extrusive effect. This can be exploited to promote overbite reduction as extrusion of posterior teeth leads to overbite reduction and can also be used for settling of the occlusion as well as antero-posterior and transverse correction pending on elastic configuration

6.2.6 Mini-Implants

Temporary anchorage devices may facilitate true anterior intrusion which may be particularly useful in adults (Polat-Ozsoy et al. 2009). The latter may potentially cope less well with increase in the vertical occlusal dimension, and extrusion may be slightly less stable in view of the absence of compensatory condylar changes in non-growing patients. Anterior mini-implant sites may be used relatively simply with direct or indirect mechanics to intrude the upper and/or lower incisors (Fig. 6.8a–e).

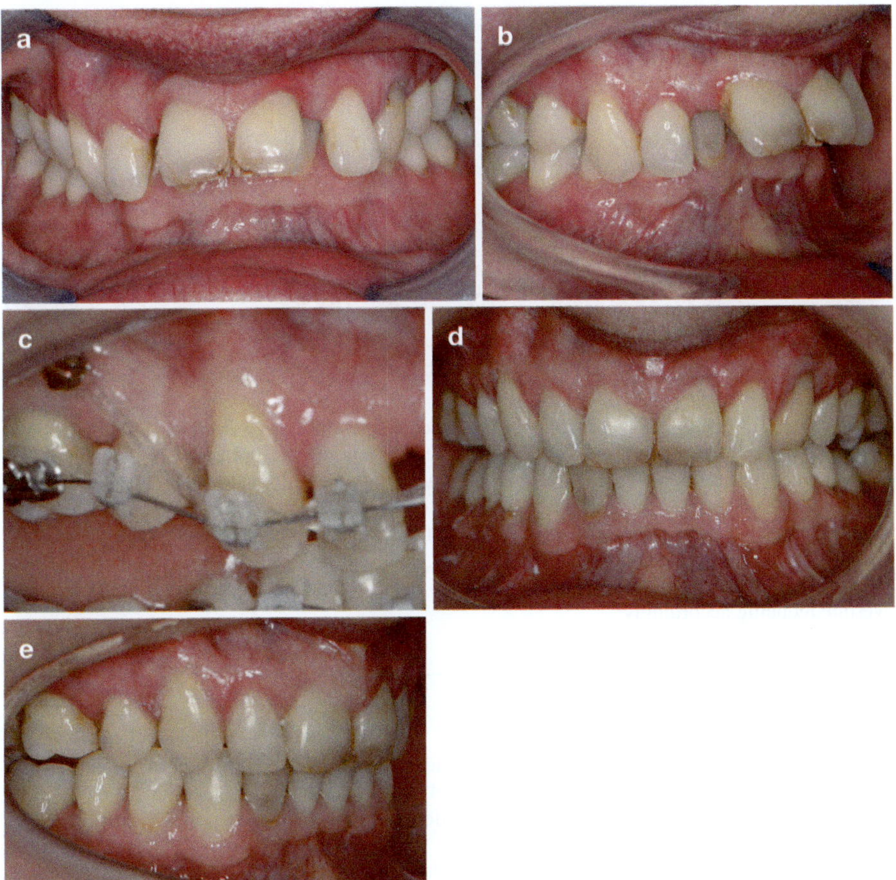

Fig. 6.8 (**a**–**e**) A deep overbite in an adult patient with a history of severe periodontitis and pathological tooth migration (**a**, **b**). Mini-implants were placed in the maxillary premolar region with light elastomeric chain to intrude the upper anteriors (**c**). A slight posterior vector also facilitated overjet reduction while a relatively vertical orientation promoted effective intrusion (**d**, **e**)

6.2.7 Intrusion Arches and Edgewise Mechanics

Established approaches to producing true intrusion include use of Ricketts and Burstone intrusion arches allied to other edgewise approaches (Fig. 6.9a–f). These techniques may require complex wire-bending skills and are used less commonly with the StraightWire appliance, particularly in view of the advent of some of the aforementioned approaches and increased use of mini-implants.

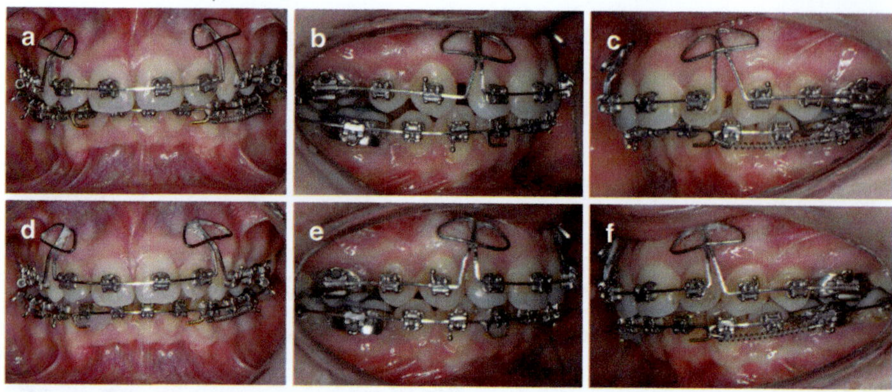

Fig. 6.9 (**a–f**) A complex Class II division 2 malocclusion with a deep overbite. Despite engagement of 0.019 × 0.025-in. stainless steel wires with reverse curves and inclusion of mandibular second molars in the appliance, the overbite was resistant (**a–c**) with the lower incisor attachments covered vertically by the upper incisors indicative of an increased overbite. Edgewise mechanics with double delta loops were fabricated (**d–f**) to facilitate space closure and intrusion with the extension mesial to the loops being more gingivally positioned than the distal segment prior to wire engagement. The vertical step is apparent following a 6-week activation period (**e**, **f**) with the overbite reducing accordingly

References

da Motta AF, de Souza MM, Bolognese AM, Guerra CJ, Mucha JN. Display of the incisors as functions of age and gender. Aust Orthod J. 2010;26(1):27.

Eberhart BB, Kuftinec MM, Baker IM. The relationship between bite depth and incisor angular change. Angle Orthod. 1990;60(1):55–8.

Kim YH. Anterior openbite and its treatment with multiloop edgewise archwire. Angle Orthod. 1987;57(4):290–321.

Kim TW, Little RM. Postretention assessment of deep overbite correction in Class II Division 2 malocclusion. Angle Orthod. 1999;69(2):175–86.

Kirschen RH, O'Higgins EA, Lee RT. The Royal London Space Planning: an integration of space analysis and treatment planning: part I: assessing the space required to meet treatment objectives. Am J Orthod Dentofac Orthop. 2000;118(4):448–55.

Mills JR. The long-term results of the proclination of lower incisors. Br Dent J. 1966;120(8):355–63.

Naini FB, Gill DS, Sharma A, Tredwin C. The aetiology, diagnosis and management of deep overbite. Dent Update. 2006;33(6):326–36.

Ng J, Major PW, Heo G, Flores-Mir C. True incisor intrusion attained during orthodontic treatment: a systematic review and meta-analysis. Am J Orthod Dentofac Orthop. 2005;128(2):212–9.

Polat-Ozsoy O, Arman-Ozcirpici A, Veziroglu F. Miniscrews for upper incisor intrusion. Eur J Orthod. 2009;31(4):412–6.

Roe P, Rungcharassaeng K, Kan JY, Patel RD, Campagni WV, Brudvik JS. The influence of upper lip length and lip mobility on maxillary incisal exposure. Am J Esthet Dent. 2012;2:116–25.

Sarver DM, Weissman SM. Nonsurgical treatment of open bite in nongrowing patients. Am J Orthod Dentofac Orthop. 1995;108(6):651–9.

Schütz-Fransson U, Bjerklin K, Lindsten R. Long-term follow-up of orthodontically treated deep bite patients. Eur J Orthod. 2006;28(5):503–12.

Selwyn-Barnett BJ. Class II/Division 2 malocclusion: a method of planning and treatment. Br J Orthod. 1996;23(1):29–36.

Space Closure

7

Orthodontic space closure usually follows overbite reduction and may accompany overjet reduction. The magnitude of space closure obviously relates to the pre-existing malocclusion, space requirements and extraction decisions. Furthermore, the degree of crowding and approach to alleviating this during earlier treatment stages has a bearing on the amount of residual space with discipline in relation to space closure and avoidance of inadvertent round tripping earlier in treatment minimising the amount of space closure required later in treatment. Conversely, where anchorage is at a premium, it may be important to preserve space early in treatment until anchorage management mechanics including inter-arch elastics can be used to direct space closure.

Sliding mechanics are typically used in contemporary StraightWire orthodontics for space closure. Either elastomeric forces (e.g. with elastomeric chain or active ligatures) or NiTi coils are used most commonly (Figs. 7.1a–c and 7.2a–e). This approach is relatively simple, does not require additional wire bending but does rely on sliding of teeth along the base wire; consequently, resistance to sliding associated with the base wire and mode of ligation are relevant. The alternative involves use of standard edgewise and loop mechanics, whereby space closing springs and complex wire formations affect space closure (Fig. 7.3a–h). With the latter, teeth do not slide along the wire, and friction has a minor bearing on space closure.

Space closure may have associated intra-arch and inter-arch effects. Intra-arch effects may include local tipping or 'dumping' of teeth into the extraction spaces. Moreover, unwanted mesiolingual rotations of posterior teeth, particularly terminal lower molars, can occur during space closure. The incisors tend to move posteriorly and extrude slightly as a consequence. This may well be beneficial pending on the occlusal presentation but can be controlled with judicious anchorage management where required. In the transverse plane, space closure tends to lead to arch constriction, particularly with second premolar or first permanent molar extraction. Arch co-ordination may therefore be required to optimise transverse dimensions and relationships.

P. Fleming, J. Seehra, *Fixed Orthodontic Appliances*, BDJ Clinician's Guides,
https://doi.org/10.1007/978-3-030-12165-5_7

Significant local intrusion and tipping of adjacent teeth can lead to the introduction of lateral open bites, particularly with use of excessive force and overly flexible base wires. While a range of mechanics can be used to address these issues, careful selection of mechanics can circumvent these side effects in the first instance.

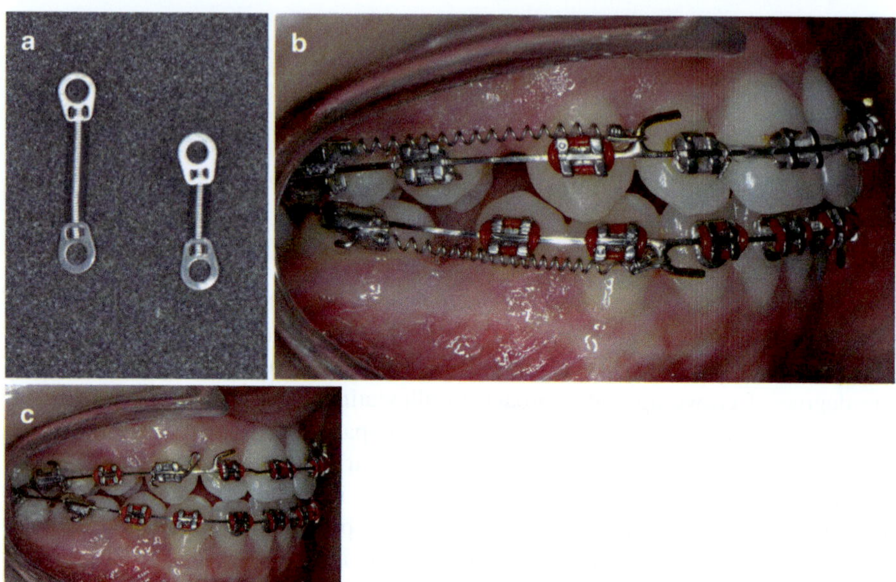

Fig. 7.1 (**a**–**c**) NiTi closing coils: 6 mm and 12 mm (**a**). Space closure in this case was facilitated with intra-arch mechanics (with NiTi closing coils) supplemented with inter-arch Class II traction to preserve Class I relationships (**b**, **c**)

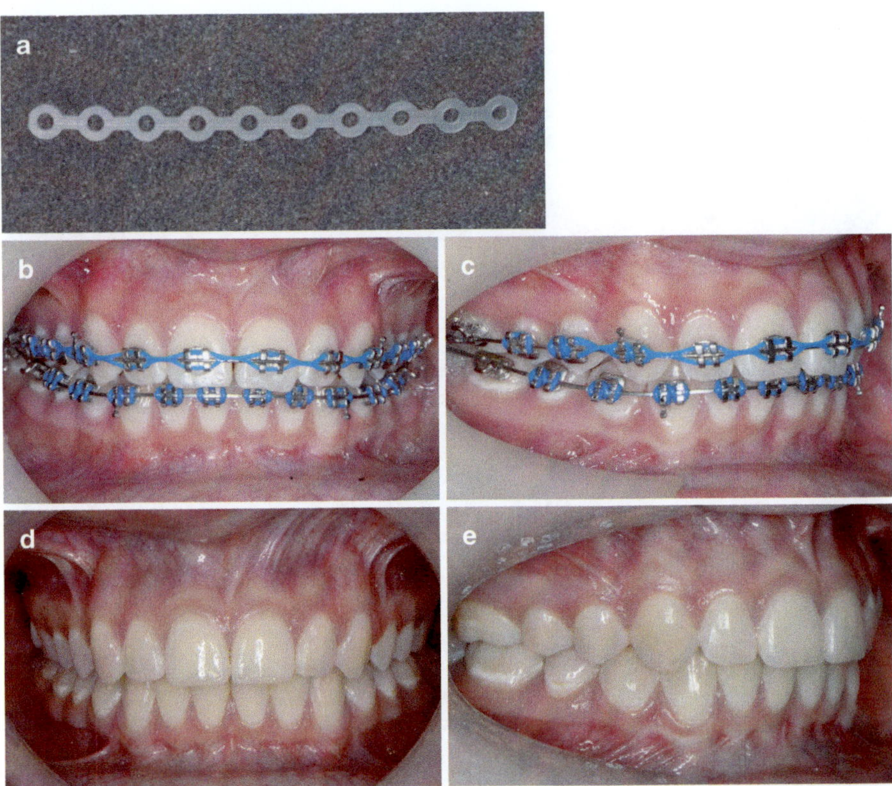

Fig. 7.2 (**a–e**) Use of elastomeric chain to close anterior spacing (**a–e**). Space was localised to the anterior regions. Space closure was therefore undertaken on round stainless steel (0.020-in.) in the first instance

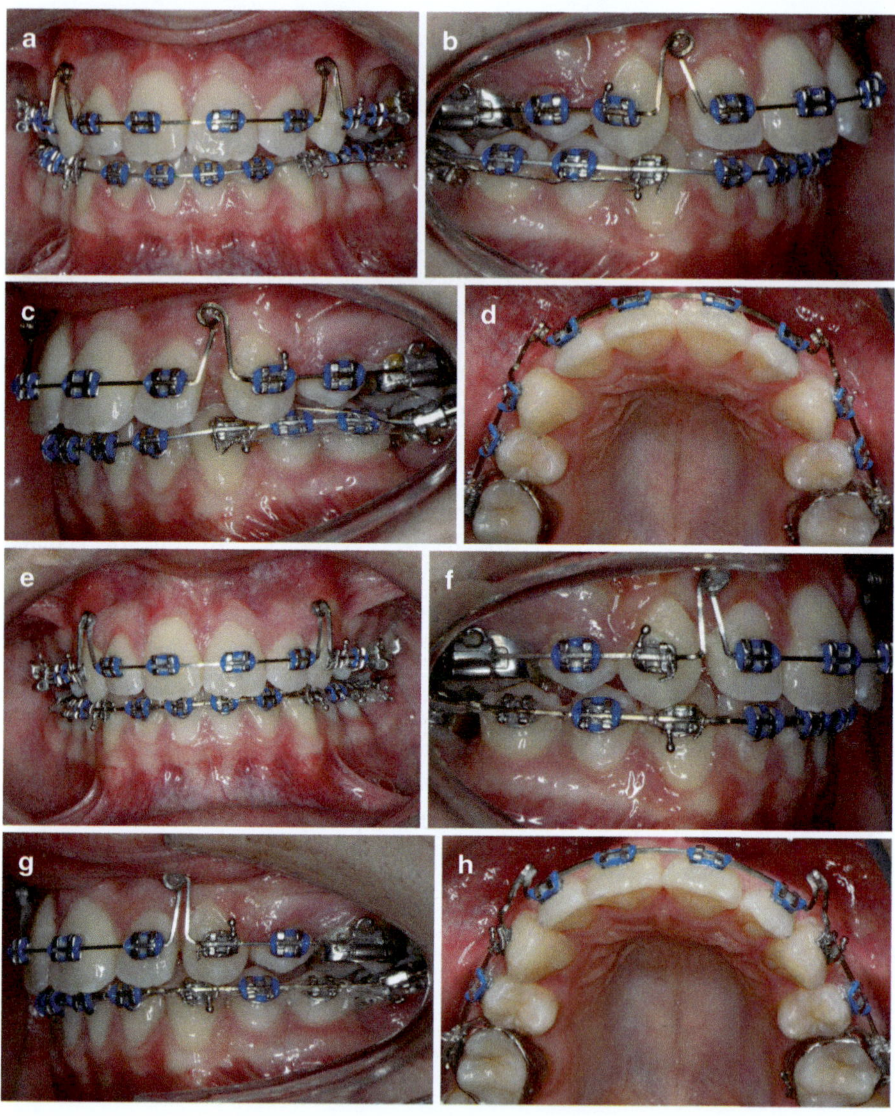

Fig. 7.3 (**a**–**h**) Edgewise closing loops formed in 0.017 × 0.025-in. stainless steel (**a**–**d**) to space close mesial to the maxillary canines. Force levels tend to be higher with this approach. Increasing wire length in the loop increases flexibility and reduces force levels accordingly

Box 7.1 Phasing of Space Closure
Where possible spacing closure is undertaken with teeth in blocks. Anterior space closure can be carried out prior to formal space closure as incisal spacing tends to be unaesthetic and can be more difficult to close. This anterior consolidation is often undertaken in intermediate wires including round steel and rectangular NiTi wires.

In the 0.022-in. slot, posterior space closure is typically carried out in 0.019 × 0.025-in. stainless steel. This wire can be engaged passively for up to 4 weeks prior to initiating space closure; however, often space closing mechanics are applied from the outset, particularly if the base wire engages relatively easily. If the anterior space has been consolidated carefully, posted wires can be placed, e.g. with brass posts tight to the distal of the lateral incisor attachments (Fig. 7.4a–j) ensuring that space closing mechanics in the posterior region will not reintroduce spacing anteriorly.

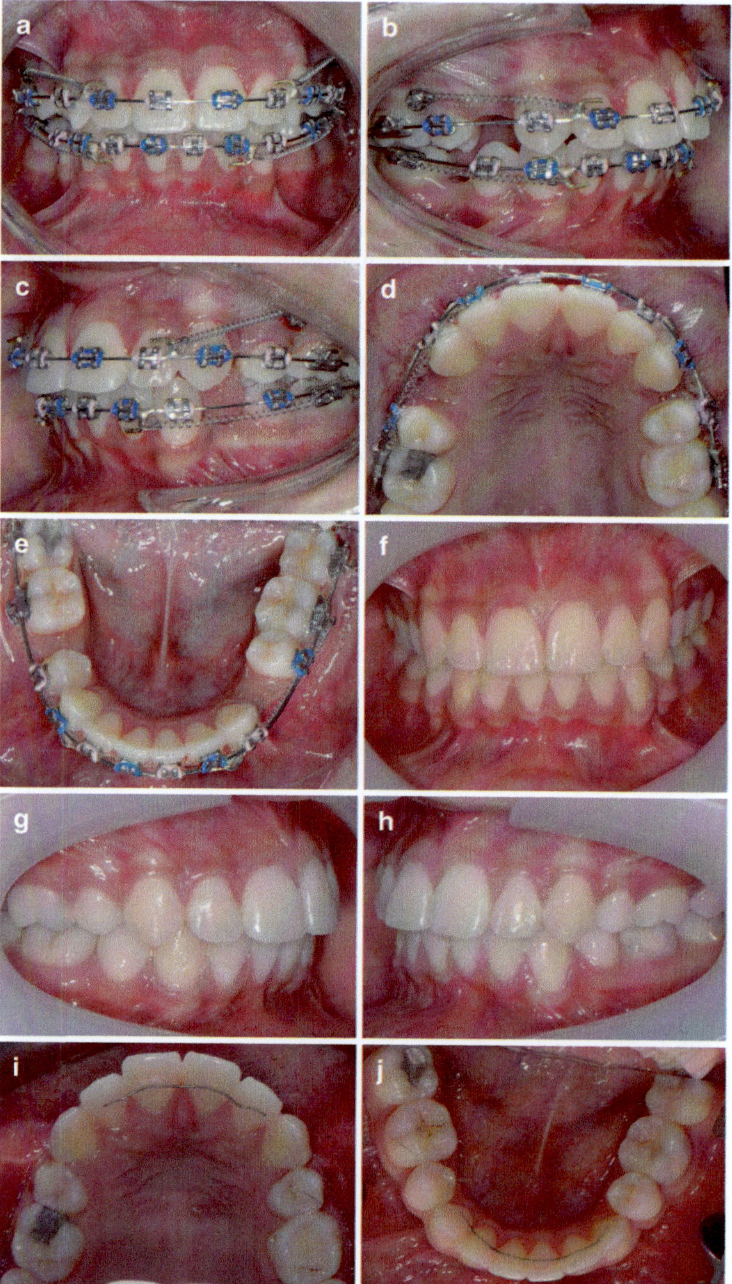

Fig. 7.4 (**a**–**j**) Space closure using NiTi closing coils in a four premolar extraction case with a significant upper midline shift. There was a significant anchorage demand on the upper right side to facilitate upper midline correction. Anchorage requirements on the upper left related to preservation of Class I relationships as the lower first premolar space was closed. Consequently, mini-implants were used to prevent posterior anchorage loss in the maxillary arch (**a**–**j**). The NiTi coils are stretched 2–3 times their original length in order to produce predictable force levels (Manhartsberger and Seidenbusch 1996) and were attached to the brass hooks on the 0.019 × 0.025-in. base wire. The brass hooks were located just distal to the lateral incisor attachments

Box 7.2 Rationale for Use of 0.019 × 0.025-In. Stainless Steel During Space Closure

A rigid base arch wire is important during space closure in order to resist the effect of active space closing mechanics. The base wire should serve a passive function of maintaining arch form and limiting possible unwanted intra-arch and inter-arch effects. 0.019 × 0.025-in. stainless steel has a low modulus of elasticity and therefore high stiffness. Stainless steel also presents a smooth surface limiting any potential resistance to sliding. Moreover, the wire is sufficiently strong to resist forces delivered by inter-arch elastics (Kusy 1997), which may be required for anchorage management. The rectangular configuration also allows for maintenance of adequate torque with significant anteroposterior changes during space closure likely to introduce retroclination of the incisors.

Despite use of rigid wires, unwanted tipping can still occur. Local variations in bracket positioning can be made to limit this with, for example, deliberate mesial angulation of first molar attachments in mandibular second premolar extraction cases and mesial angulation of second molar attachments to mitigate against mesial tipping of these teeth during first molar extraction space closure.

In certain circumstances, undersized (0.017 × 0.025-in.) or round (0.018- or 0.020-in.) stainless steel can be used where inclination changes of the labial segments are required. In particular, full torque expression in the lower anterior region may be undesirable in Class III cases where preferential retraction of the mandibular incisors may be required in order to establish an increased overjet and overbite (Fig. 7.5a–f).

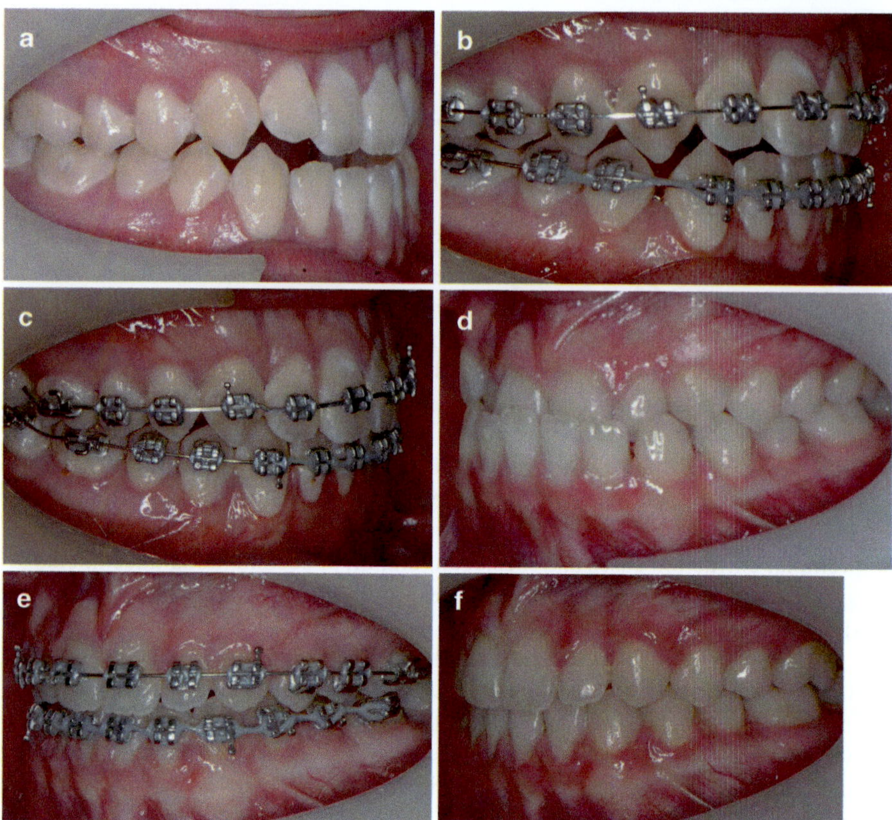

Fig. 7.5 (**a**–**f**) Space closure with elastomeric chain in the lower arch in Class III camouflage. The mandibular canine bracket has been reversed to promote distal crown tipping and mandibular incisor retraction (**a**, **b**). A round (0.018-in.) stainless steel wire has been placed to encourage retroclination of the mandibular incisors in order to establish a positive overjet. A vertical offset has been placed in the upper 0.019 × 0.025-in. TMA finishing wire to increase the overbite (**c**). A similar approach with round 0.018-in. steel in the lower arch allowing the lower incisors to retrocline during space closure (**d**–**f**). Full torque expression can be undertaken once a positive overjet and overbite have been obtained

Box 7.3 Elastomeric Chain or NiTi Coils?

A number of randomised controlled trials have been carried out evaluating the relative merits of NiTi closing coils and elastomeric alternatives. Dixon et al. (2002) reported a mean rate of space closure of 0.81 mm per month with NiTi coils versus 0.58 mm with elastomeric chain and 0.35 with active elastomeric ligatures. Similarly, Samuels et al. (1993) reported improved efficiency and consistency with NiTi coils. Elastomeric chain does, however, also offer a predictable means of space closure and is more versatile in that anterior space closure can also be undertaken in a simple manner in concert with posterior space closure (Figs. 7.6a–h and 7.7a–i).

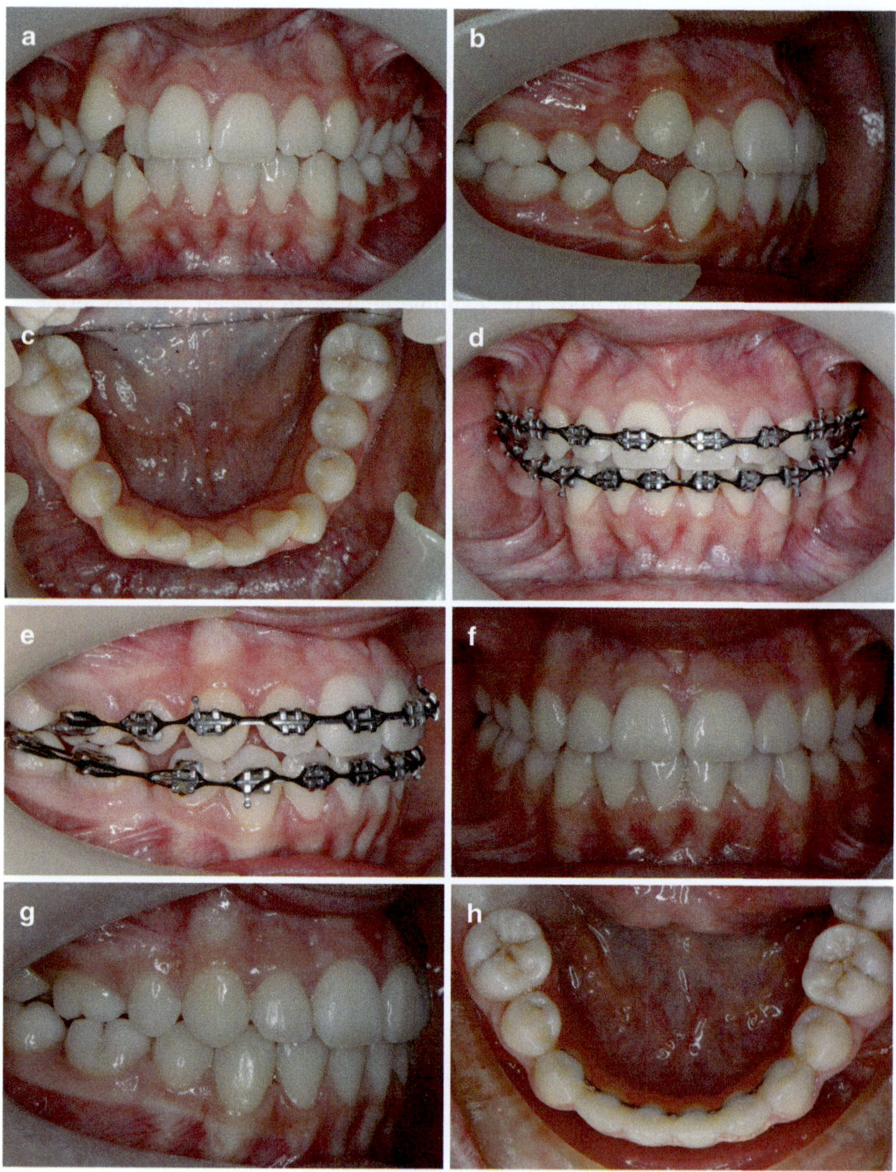

Fig. 7.6 (**a**–**h**) A Class I malocclusion with dual-arch crowding treated with loss of four premolar units. Space closure is undertaken with elastomeric chain in this instance as there is space in the lower anterior region (**a**–**c**). Note that the elastomeric chain has been extended to the mandibular second molar (**d**, **e**). This may risk inducing mesiolingual rotation of this tooth; elastomeric chain should therefore not be applied to the terminal bonded tooth in the lower appliance where possible. Space closure was completed efficiently with preservation of Class I relationships and complete midline correction (**f**–**h**)

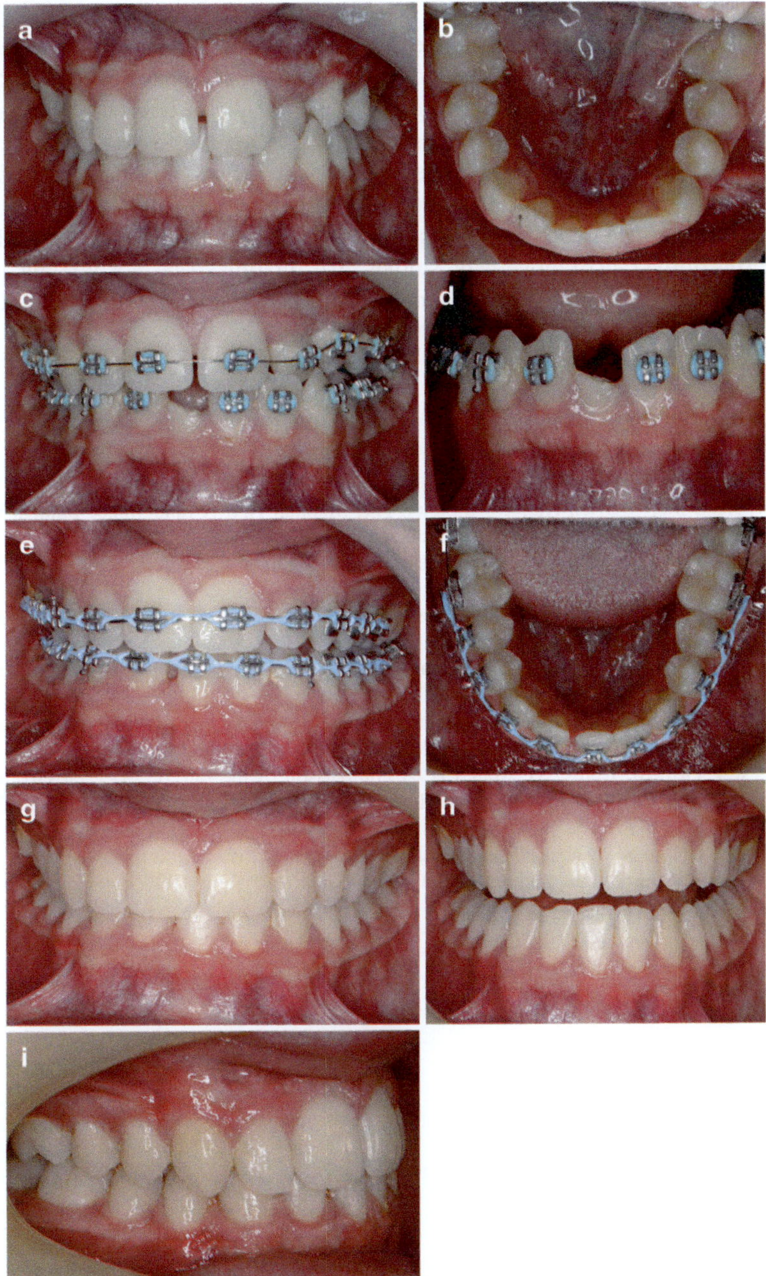

Fig. 7.7 (**a**–**i**) A complex Class I malocclusion involved previous loss of an ectopic maxillary left canine and localised crossbites (**a**, **b**). Non-extraction-based treatment had been planned with transverse co-ordination; however, trauma was sustained to the lower anteriors with the lower right central incisor fractured at gingival level (**c**, **d**). A decision was made to space close following loss of the lower incisor with lower arch constriction facilitating crossbite correction. Elastomeric chain was placed in both arches to produce both anterior and posterior space closure (**e**, **f**). Complete space closure was achieved with improved transverse co-ordination and good buccal segment interdigitation (**g**–**i**)

Box 7.4 Force Levels and Rate of Space Closure

The optimal force level required for tooth movement remains unclear (Ren et al. 2003). Samuels et al. (1998) reported no benefit associated with forces in excess of 150 g during space closure. However, space closure is a process, and it is likely that the force required to initiate tooth movement might differ from that required to continue movement during the process. Typically, reactivation of space closure mechanics is undertaken at intervals of 4–10 weeks. In terms of the rate of movement, studies investigating space closure typically report rates of no more than 1 mm per month or less (Dixon et al. 2002; Nightingale and Jones 2003).

References

Dixon V, Read MJ, O Brien KD, Worthington HV, Mandall NA. A randomized clinical trial to compare three methods of orthodontic space closure. J Orthod. 2002;29(1):31–6.

Kusy RP. A review of contemporary archwires: their properties and characteristics. Angle Orthod. 1997;67(3):197–207.

Manhartsberger C, Seidenbusch W. Force delivery of Ni-Ti coil springs. Am J Orthod Dentofac Orthop. 1996;109(1):8–21.

Nightingale C, Jones SP. A clinical investigation of force delivery systems for orthodontic space closure. J Orthod. 2003;30(3):229–36.

Ren Y, Maltha JC, Kuijpers-Jagtman AM. Optimum force magnitude for orthodontic tooth movement: a systematic literature review. Angle Orthod. 2003;73(1):86–92.

Samuels RH, Orth M, Rudge SJ, Mair LH. A comparison of the rate of space closure using a nickel-titanium spring and an elastic module: a clinical study. Am J Orthod Dentofac Orthop. 1993;103(5):464–7.

Samuels RH, Rudge SJ, Mair LH. A clinical study of space closure with nickel-titanium closed coil springs and an elastic module. Am J Orthod Dentofac Orthop. 1998;114(1):73–9.

8 Finishing Stages

The finishing stage of treatment generally involves detailing the overall occlusion and individual tooth position prior to removing the fixed appliance. It tends to follow space closure in extraction cases, may involve preservation of any space closure and incorporates completion of intra-arch and inter-arch objectives. This stage of treatment may span anything from a matter of weeks to a number of months with more time-consuming finishing changes including torque correction, while other alignment and vertical changes tend to improve more rapidly.

The finishing stage may involve a combination of different arch wires, pending on the objectives and the need for repositioning of brackets, torque correction, use of intra-oral elastics and wire bending. The degree of finishing required and indeed feasible is influenced by multiple factors including the planned treatment aims and objectives, the mechanics employed, the chosen appliance, patient compliance during treatment, critically the initial bracket positioning (Poling 1999), and the degree to which any imperfections were dealt with during earlier phases.

When assessing the degree and nature of finishing required, intra-arch and inter-arch occlusal features should be evaluated in all three dimensions. To achieve an optimal result in accordance with the planned treatment aims and objectives, each dental arch should be inspected in detail individually and with the teeth in occlusion. Within each arch, all spaces should be closed, rotations and vertical issues addressed with the upper and lower incisors at the correct angulation and inclination. In occlusion, the impact of any posterior vertical intra-arch discrepancies (marginal ridge height discrepancies) on the occlusion is evaluated. The arches should be co-ordinated transversely without crossbites or associated displacements with good buccal segment interdigitation (Poling 1999).

Optimal finishing of a case will typically require a degree of wire bending which is outlined in Chap. 9. Historically, a panoramic radiograph has been used as a diagnostic aid to evaluate the alignment of the anterior and posterior dentition providing information in relation to the angulation of the teeth, in particular. However, the merit of this has been contested with this view shown to be accurate (to within 2.5°)

P. Fleming, J. Seehra, *Fixed Orthodontic Appliances*, BDJ Clinician's Guides,
https://doi.org/10.1007/978-3-030-12165-5_8

in just 26% of instances, with upper canine-first premolar roots being projected as more divergent and lower lateral incisor-canine appearing more convergent radiographically (Owens and Johal 2008).

The practical steps involved in the placement of elastics and keeping spaces closed during the finishing stage are outlined below.

Box 8.1 Ideal Static and Dynamic Occlusion
Based on 120 study models of untreated patients who were deemed to have the 'ideal occlusion', the six keys to a normal occlusion were proposed (Andrews 1972). Although a common treatment objective is to deliver an ideal 'Andrews' six keys' occlusion (Chap. 1), it is established that optimal occlusal outcomes are not routinely achieved regardless of the bracket prescription used.

The functional or dynamic occlusion should also be considered. The ideal dynamic relationships are unclear, and the relevance of the dynamic occlusal relationships in an unrestored, healthy dentition is debated. Bilateral contacts in retruded contact position (RCP) are considered optimal with working side contacts between teeth during lateral excursions (canine guidance or group function) and no contacts on the nonworking side during lateral excursions a reasonable objective (Clark and Evans 2001) (Fig. 8.1a, b).

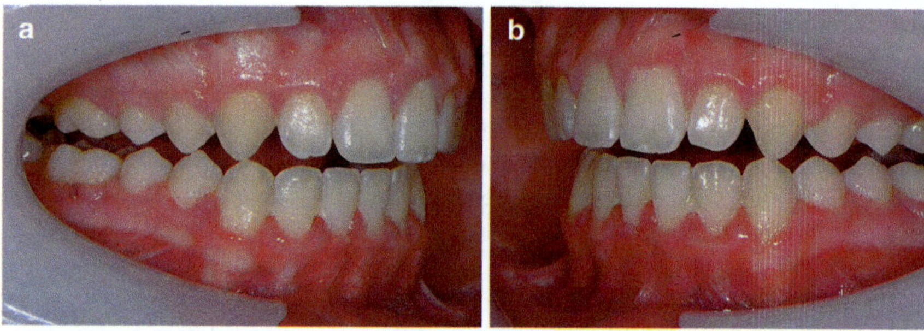

Fig. 8.1 (**a**, **b**) Canine guidance on lateral excursions with posterior disclusion

Box 8.2 Ideal Properties of an Archwire Used for Finishing Stages of Treatment
Ideally, archwires used for finishing stages of treatment including wire bending should facilitate space closure and maintenance of the arch form and allow differential tooth movements (first, second and third order) (Chap. 9). The selected archwires should typically exhibit the following properties: low friction, formability, high stiffness and low range. However, high friction may be helpful where torque requirements are high.

Common archwires used in this phase of treatment are rectangular braided stainless steel (0.019 × 0.025 in.) (Fig. 8.2a), rectangular Beta-Titanium (0.019 × 0.025-in. TMA) (Fig. 8.2b) and round stainless steel (0.018 in.) (Fig. 8.2c). Specifically, rectangular braided steel offers the benefit of maintaining third order (torque) control while providing the flexibility to allow for occlusal settling and some formability to place local bends. Similarly, Beta-Titanium (or Titanium-Molybdenum alloy) can be used where torque is required and formability is important as it is slightly more flexible than stainless steel and can be used for artistic finishing bends with lower force levels than comparable stainless steel wires. Round stainless steel again provides the advantage of formability, low resistance to sliding and arch form control but does lack three-dimensional control.

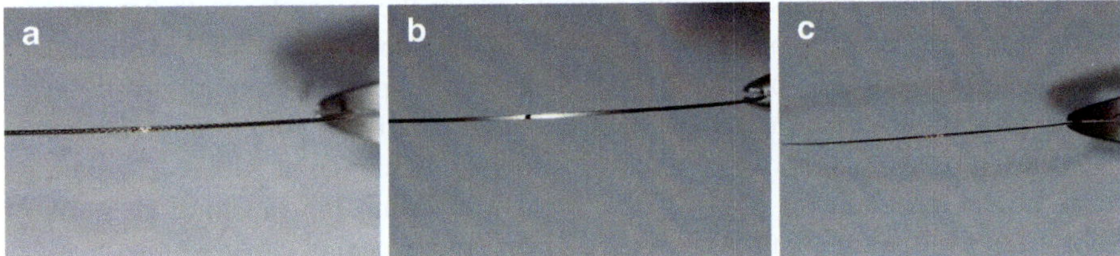

Fig. 8.2 (**a–c**) Possible finishing archwires including: rectangular braided stainless steel (0.019 × 0.025 in.) (**a**) rectangular Beta-Titanium (0.019 × 0.025-in. TMA) (**b**) and round stainless steel (0.018 in.) (**c**)

Box 8.3 Repositioning of Brackets to Correct Errors in Bracket Position

Errors in bracket positioning are a common cause of variation in tooth position during fixed appliance treatment. It is important to critically review the position of the brackets during the initial alignment phase (Chap. 4). Location should be assessed in relation to the ideal position from both the buccal aspect and vertically using the long axis of the tooth as a reference guide (Chap. 3). Early identification of bracket position errors and repositioning may obviate the need for complex wire bending during finishing stages and possible extension of treatment.

Horizontal bracket positioning errors result in a rotational discrepancy (first order). This occurs commonly in the lower canine and lateral incisor region (Fig. 8.3a), whereby the bracket is positioned distal to the ideal position on the lower canine. To correct this the lower canine bracket can be repositioned slightly mesial to the long axis of the crown and a round Nickel-Titanium archwire ligated (Fig. 8.3b). Alternatively, a derotation (first order) bend can be placed in a round (0.018-in.) stainless steel wire to correct rotations (Fig. 8.4a–d).

An angulation error can lead to incorrect crown positioning in the mesio-distal plane relative to the root but also residual spacing within the arch and a failure to achieve the ideal anterior and/or posterior occlusion (Fig. 8.5a–c). An abnormal crown morphology can also lead to non-ideal bracket positioning and resultant first, second or third order issues (Fig. 8.6a–d).

Vertical bracket position errors can result in third order tooth errors (Miethke and Melsen 1999). Even minor changes up to 1 mm in the vertical dimension can result in a 10-degree change in inclination (torque) (Fig. 8.7a, b: black lines). Vertical errors can also manifest in the buccal segments. A common error is incorrect placement of premolar brackets. In particular, iatrogenic occlusal positioning of second premolar brackets can lead to slight intrusion of these teeth relative to adjacent premolars and first molars. Marginal ridge discrepancies between the premolar and first permanent molar and incomplete interdigitation of the occlusion therefore result (Fig. 8.8a). This commonly occurs in young patients where the premolar teeth have not fully erupted and the brackets are placed in the centre of the visible clinical crown. To avoid this, premolar brackets should be placed more gingivally at the initial bond-up stage (Chap. 3). However, repositioning of premolar brackets in a more gingival position and use of round or rectangular Nickel-Titanium archwires can help to improve the occlusion during the finishing stage. A posterior box elastic can also be used to seat the buccal occlusion more positively, particularly where more general settling is required (Fig. 8.8b, c). Localised extrusion bends (Chap. 9) can also be placed in formable wires (e.g. stainless steel or TMA) to improve the vertical position of the premolar teeth, correcting marginal ridge discrepancy and settling the occlusion. To improve the vertical position of the UL5, an extrusion bend was placed to establish contact with opposing teeth and optimal buccal interdigitation (Fig. 8.9a–c).

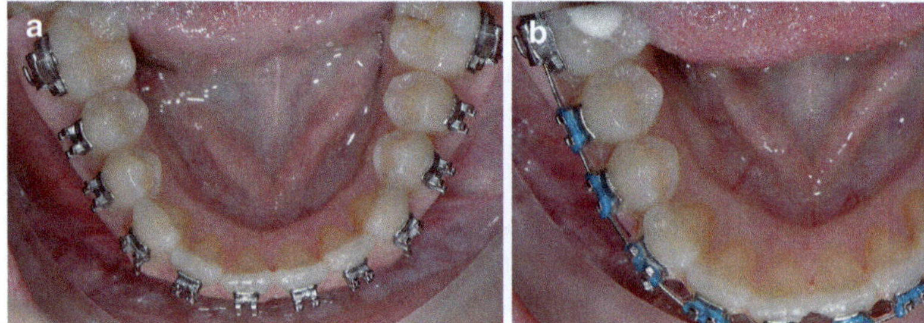

Fig. 8.3 (**a**, **b**) Horizontal bracket positioning error on the lower right canine with iatrogenic distal positioning leading to contact point slippage (**a**). This was corrected with repositioning (**b**)

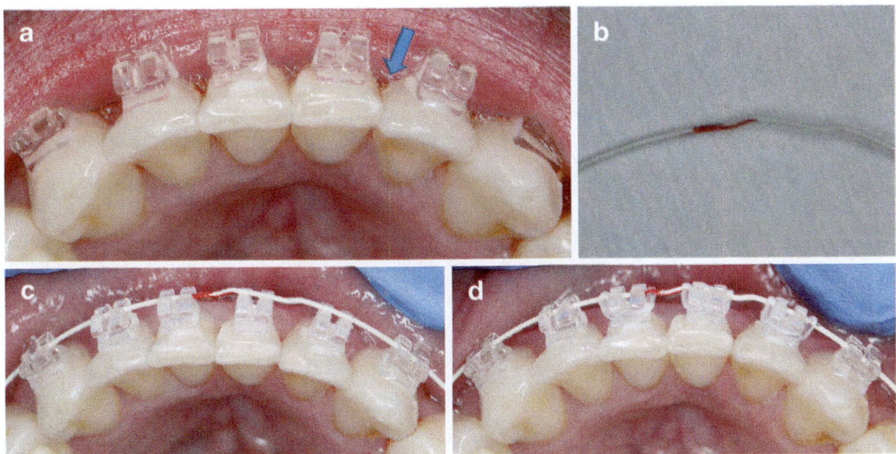

Fig. 8.4 (**a**–**d**) An error in bracket positioning (LR1) has resulted in a rotational discrepancy between the LR1 and LR2 (**a**). A first order bend is placed in a round 0.018-in. stainless steel wire to correct (**b**). The archwire is ligated fully into the bracket slot leading to correction (**c**, **d**)

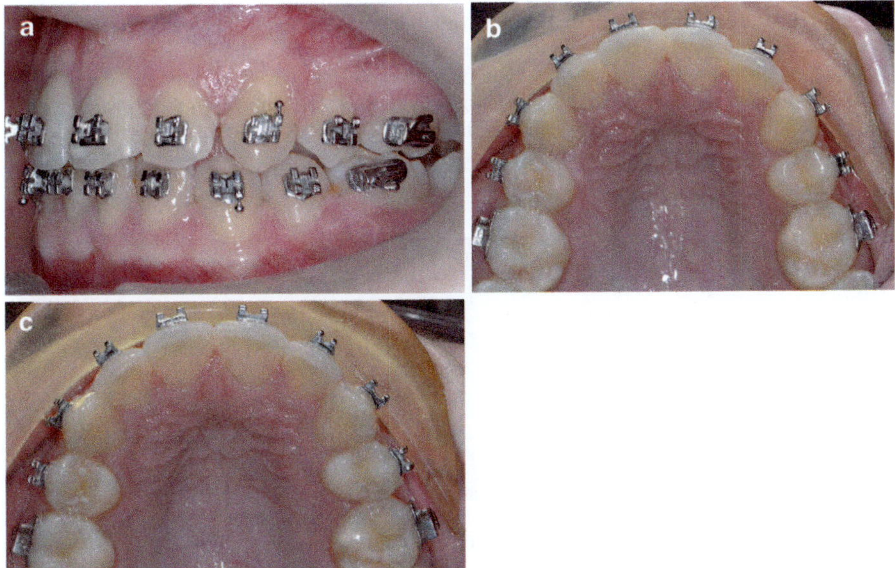

Fig. 8.5 (**a**–**c**) The maxillary left lateral incisor is mesially angulated due to imperfect bracket positioning (**a**, **b**). Repositioning of the UL2 bracket results in correction of the root position, allows for subsequent space closure and improved occlusion (**c**)

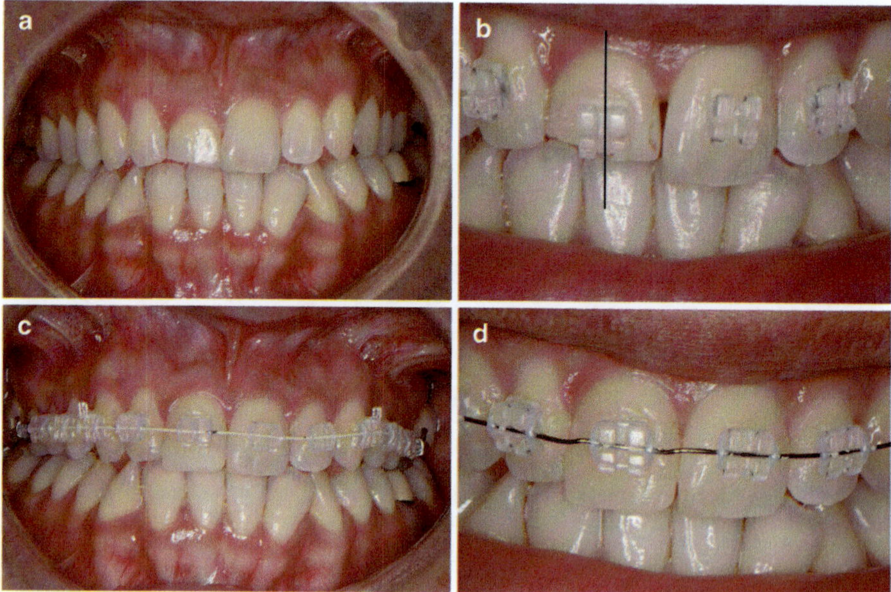

Fig. 8.6 (**a–d**) The incisal fracture associated with the UR1 resulted in an angulation error which was corrected with an angulation (second order) bend to tip the root mesially towards the end of treatment (**a–d**). An initial NiTi aligning wire was placed as close to the LA point as possible to permit intrusion of the teeth and associated gingival harmony (**a–c**); however, the crown remained mesially angulated necessitating a distal angulation bend in 0.018-in. stainless steel (**d**) to move the crown distally relative to the root position

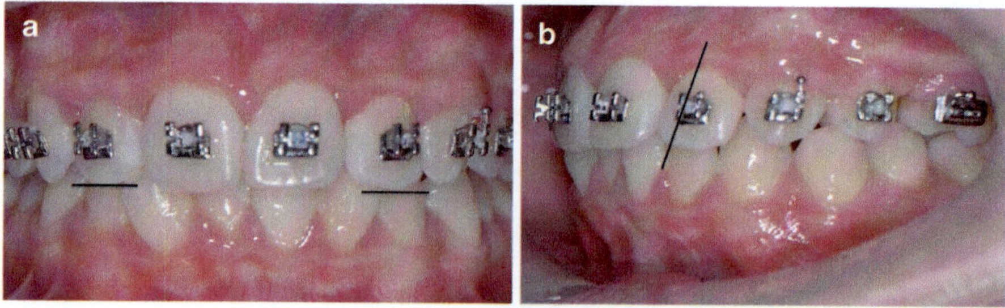

Fig. 8.7 (**a, b**) Incorrect vertical positioning of the lateral incisor brackets contributes to torque change

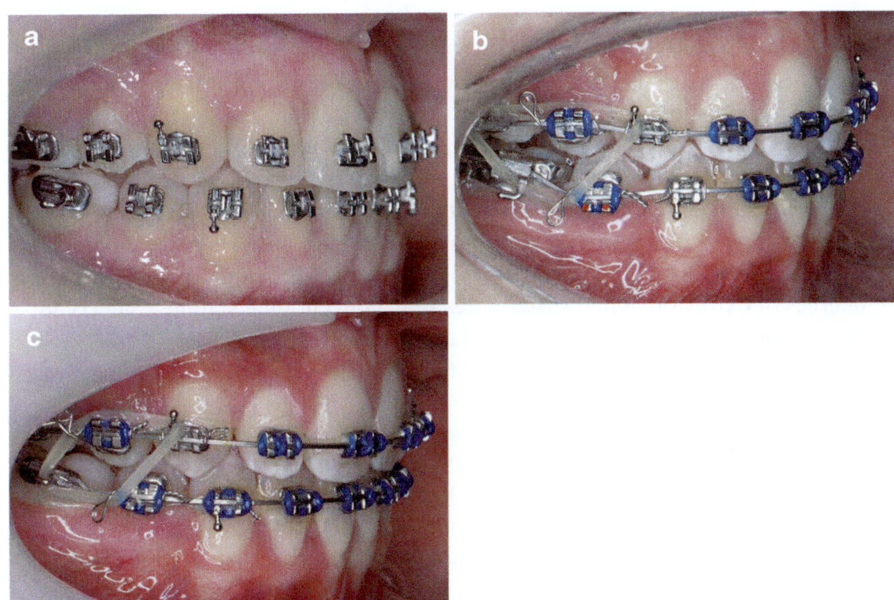

Fig. 8.8 (**a–c**) Incorrect positioning of first premolar brackets leading to local open bites. Correction of the bracket position with engagement of NiTi wires resulted in correction of intra- and inter- arch features

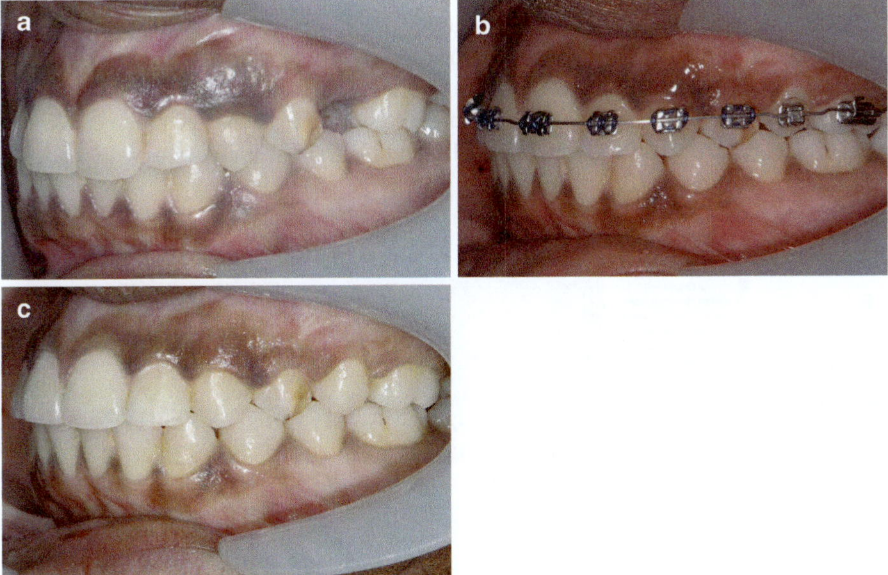

Fig. 8.9 (**a–c**) An extrusion bend was required to finalise the position of the second premolar. This is performed in 0.018-inch SS

Box 8.4 Use of Elastics

Intra-oral elastics or intermaxillary elastics can be used in various combinations during the finishing stage to improve the occlusion in the antero-posterior, vertical and transverse dimensions (Fig. 8.10a). To optimise buccal segment interdigitation, a combination of wires including rectangular braided stainless steel (Fig. 8.10b, c), conventional stainless steel, NiTi or Beta-Titanium (Fig. 8.10d, e) with settling elastics can be used. More flexible wires including NiTi or braided steel are recommended for arches which might require greater degrees of extrusion, while stiffer wires (e.g. conventional stainless steel) can be used in an opposing arch if less relative movement is needed.

Placement of an anterior box elastic can help to extrude the upper and lower labial segments and increase the overbite (Fig. 8.11a, b). Again, preferential extrusion within a single arch can be promoted with use of more flexible base wires in this arch. Elastics can be retained using hooks on attachments (typically canines and molars), on arch wire hooks, or with steel Kobayashi ligatures where required. During the final stages of space closure, the use of intermaxillary elastics in the antero-posterior dimension such as Class II elastics can help to reinforce the anchorage (Fig. 8.12a, b) but also improve the buccal segment relationship (Fig. 8.12c, d).

Centreline correction during the final stages of space closure and during finishing can be facilitated with the use of intermaxillary elastics. In the absence of a skeletal asymmetry, tooth size discrepancy or significant tip or torque problem, most centreline deviations can be attributed to asymmetric buccal segment relationships precipitated by anchorage loss or the dictates of the presenting occlusion. In Fig. 8.13a, b the dental centrelines are noncoincident due to the Class II buccal relationship on the left side and Class III buccal relationship on the right. This was addressed with the use of asymmetric elastics: Class II (left side) and Class III (right side) in conjuction with good patient compliance (Fig. 8.13c–f).

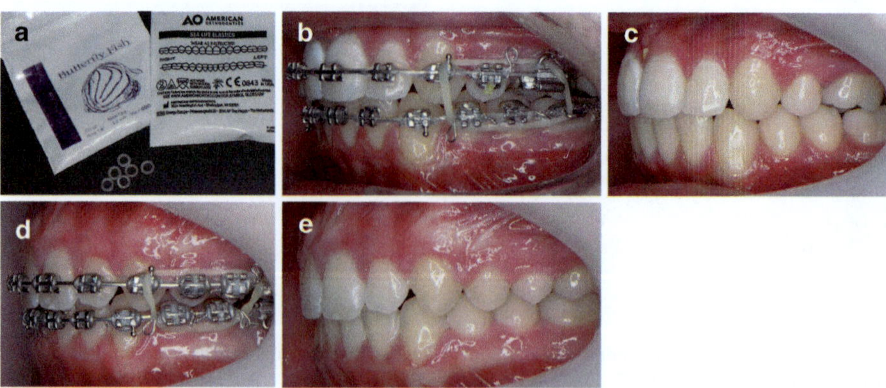

Fig. 8.10 (**a**–**e**) Intermaxillary elastics to settle the posterior occlusion. The use of more flexible wires including NiTi or braided steel can promote more effective extrusion and seating of the occlusion

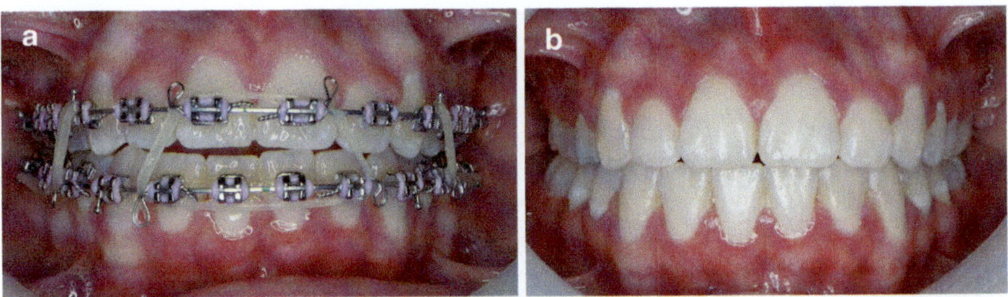

Fig. 8.11 (**a**, **b**) Use of anterior box elastic can help to extrude the upper and lower anteriors improving the overbite

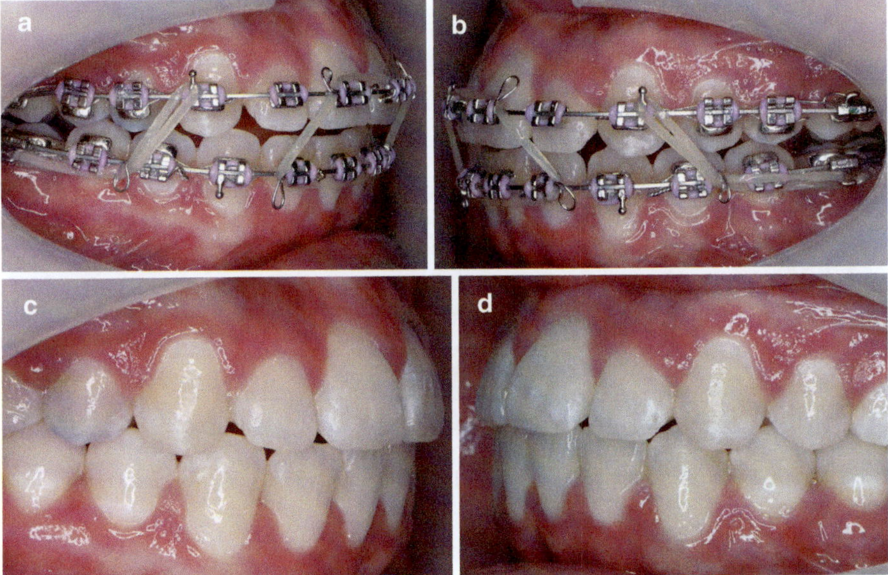

Fig. 8.12 (**a**–**d**) A combination of anterior and posterior elastics to improve Class II relationships and increase the overbite. Use of posterior elastics, in isolation, risks exacerbating the open bite tendency. Anterior elastics are typically recommended for nights-only wear

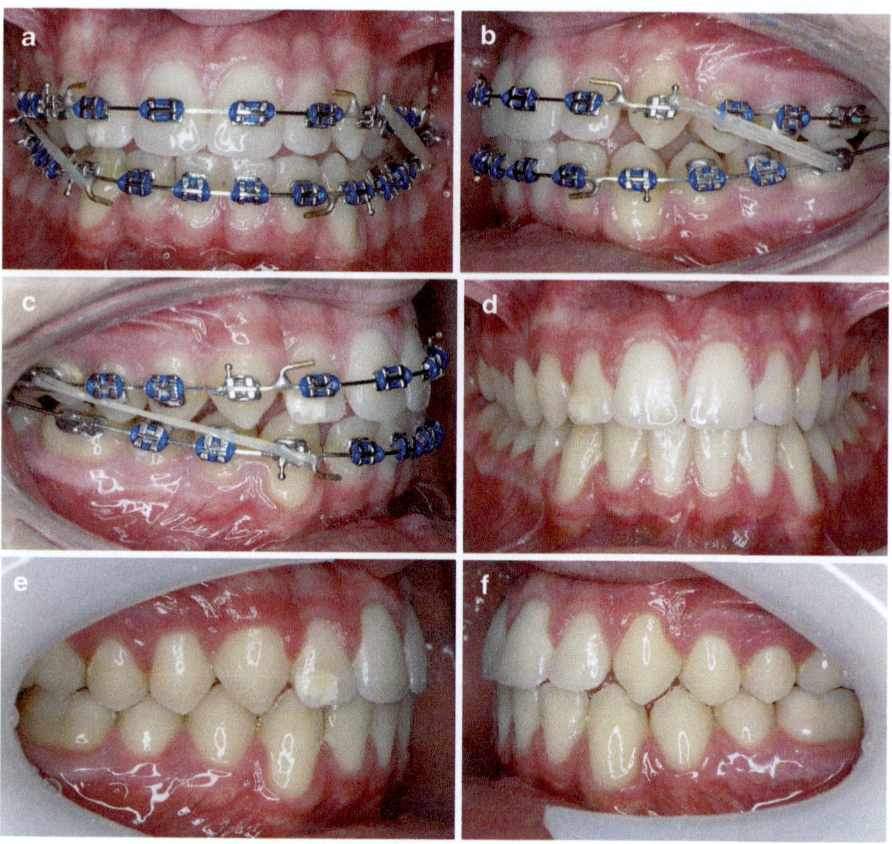

Fig. 8.13 (**a**–**f**) Use of asymmetric posterior elastics to improve the occlusion and promote midline correction

Box 8.5 Managing a Tooth Size Discrepancy

A microdont tooth is regarded as one more than two standard deviations smaller than the average width. Tooth size discrepancies should be identified at the treatment planning stage and the appropriate management planned in relation to possible need for build-up or compensatory tooth size reduction in the opposing arch or quadrant to maintain optimal intra-arch and inter-arch relationships. Commonly, a discrepancy is found in the upper arch involving the upper lateral incisors (Fig. 8.14a–c). During the finishing stages, this may manifest as residual spaces adjacent to the lateral incisors despite the presence of a good fit of the buccal segments, average overbite and overjet. Alternatively, if space closure is possible, a reduced overjet and overbite may result in view of the reduced volume of upper anterior tooth tissue. Residual maxillary arch space can be managed by adding composite restorations to increase the dimension of the lateral incisors. Increasing the inclination (torque) of the upper incisors by wire bending (Chap. 9) may also help the upper incisors occupy more space and assist with closure of residual spaces. Alternatively, by carrying out interproximal reduction of the lower labial segment (Fig. 8.14d–f) followed by space closure in the upper arch (Fig. 8.14g–i), closure of the residual space can be achieved without the need for composite additions (Fig. 8.14j).

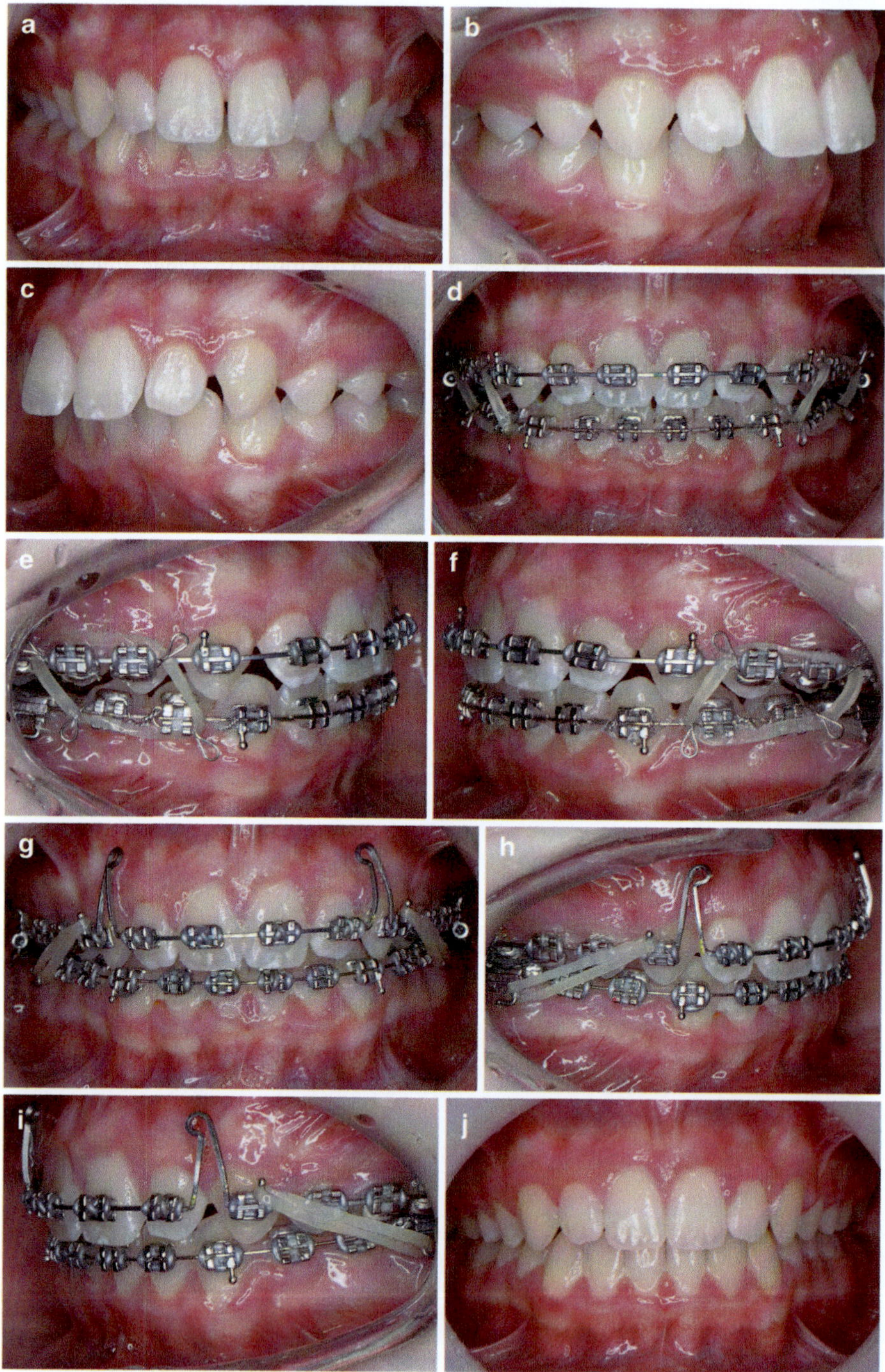

Fig. 8.14 (**a–j**) Diminutive maxillary lateral incisors compensated for with light lower inter-proximal reduction with use of Sandusky closing loops (**g–i**) to complete space closure

8.1 Orthodontic Finishing: Practical Steps

Spaces can be kept closed in a variety of ways during the finishing stage. The simplest approach is to cinch the distal ends of the wire tightly behind the terminal attachments to mitigate against unwanted arch lengthening. This approach obviates the need for further auxiliaries and associated implications in relation to risk of breakage and plaque accumulation.

Alternatively, a long stainless steel ligature can be used in two configurations (underneath or above the archwire). Firstly, similar to a laceback, an undertie can be placed around the brackets. The ligature is placed above and below the gingival and occlusal aspects of the brackets. The ends of the long ligature are brought together with either a mosquito forceps or Mathieu ligature pliers (Chap. 2), twisted and cut off using a ligature cutter instrument leaving approx. 3 mm of a ligature end. The remaining end of the undertie is then tucked away from the soft tissues using a ligature director. The archwire is then ligated in the conventional manner (Fig. 8.15a–h).

An overtie can also be placed. With the archwire in place, a ligature is placed above and below the gingival and occlusal aspects of the first bracket. The ends of the long ligature are brought together with either a mosquito forceps or Mathieu ligature pliers (Chap. 2) and twisted together before the next bracket. The process is

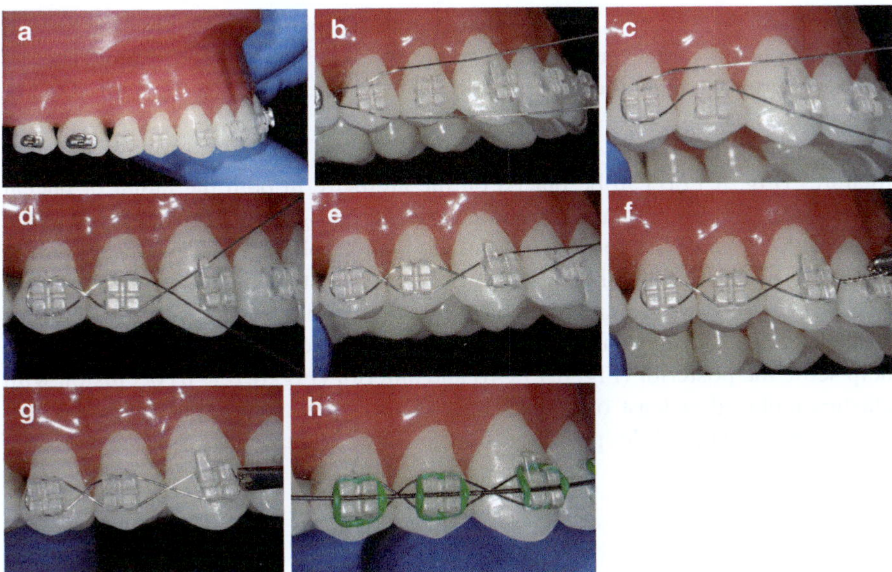

Fig. 8.15 (**a**–**h**). Placement of a stainless steel ligature as an undertie to keep space closed during the finishing stage

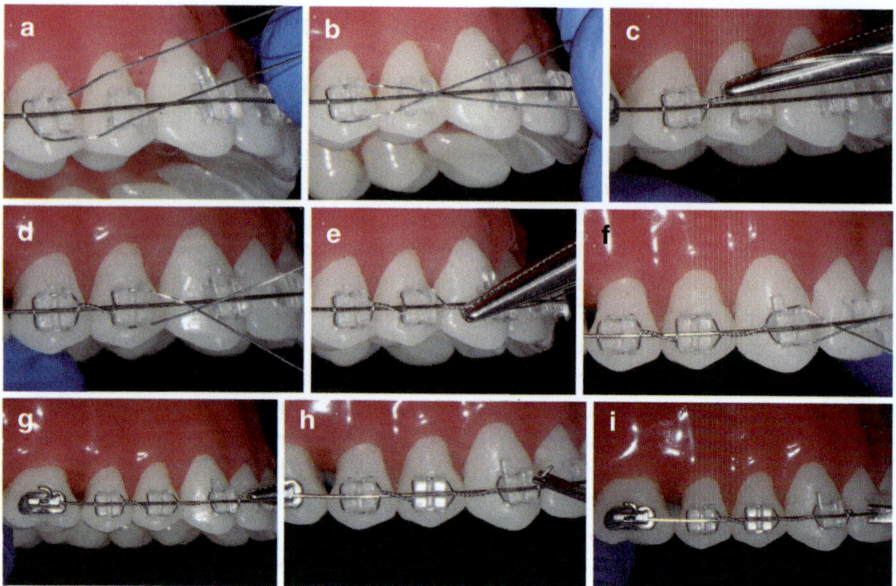

Fig. 8.16 (**a–i**). Placement of a stainless steel ligature as an overtie to keep space closed during the finishing stage

repeated, and the final ends of the long ligature are brought together twisted and cut off using a ligature cutter instrument leaving approx. 3 mm of the ligature. The tail of the overtie is then tucked from the soft tissues using a ligature director (Fig. 8.16a–i).

To facilitate the use of intermaxillary elastics for vertical settling, Kobayashi ligatures (Fig. 8.17a) can be placed on the archwire in both the labial or buccal segments. They can be placed over the elastomeric ligature to improve retention. Using either a mosquito forceps or Mathieu ligature pliers, the Kobayashi ligature is placed around the bracket, twisted tightly and cut off using a ligature cutter (Fig. 8.17b–g). Patients can be instructed on correct placement of settling elastics around the Kobayashi ligatures and the hooks on fixed appliance attachments to help settle the posterior (Fig. 8.19a–h) and anterior (Fig. 8.18a–h) occlusion with elastics replaced at least once daily and anterior elastics normally reserved for nights-only wear, while posterior elastics are amenable to full-time use, if required.

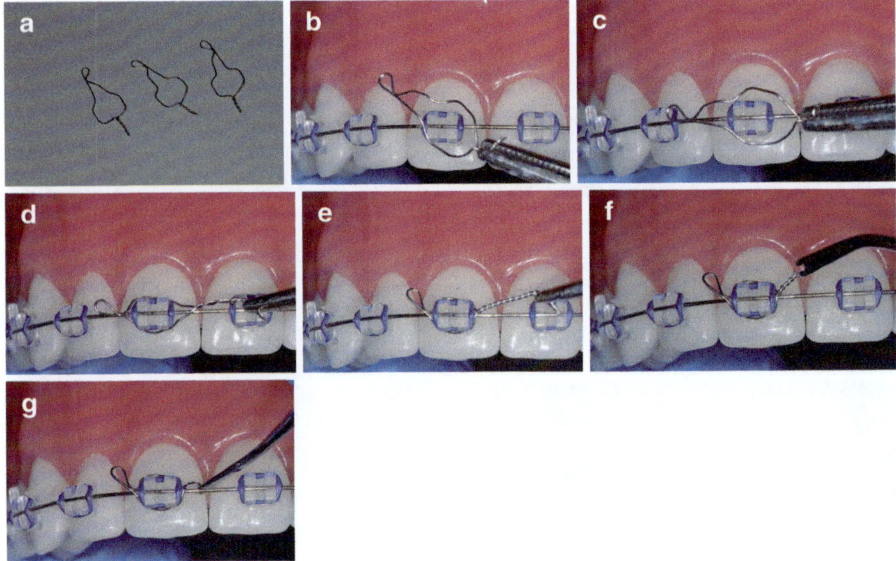

Fig. 8.17 (**a–g**) A Kobayashi ligature placed on the maxillary right central incisor

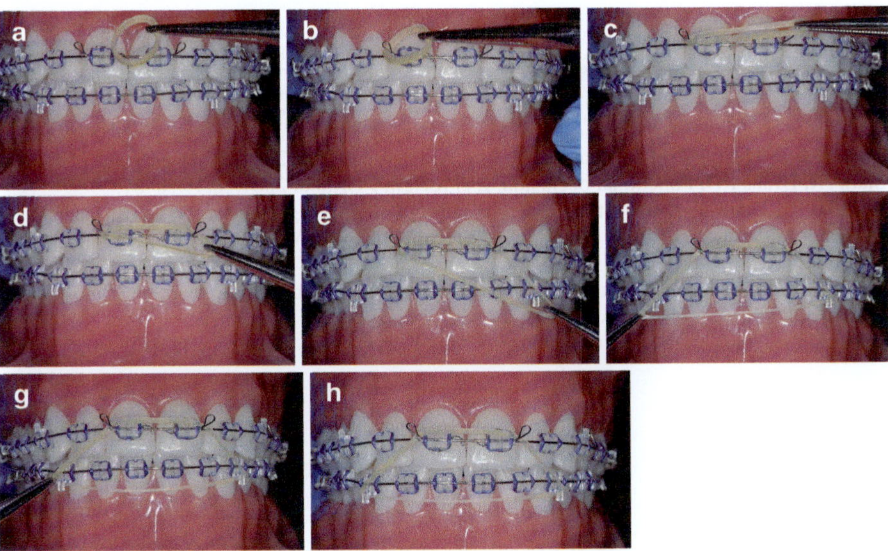

Fig. 8.18 (**a–h**) An anterior box elastic extending from the maxillary central incisors to the mandibular canines

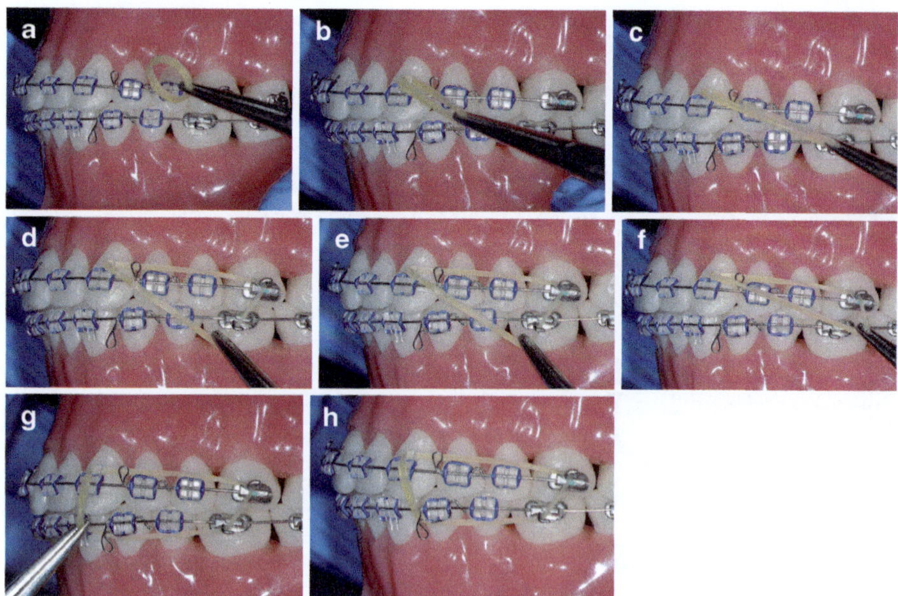

Fig. 8.19 (**a–h**) A posterior box elastic extending from the maxillary canines and first molars to the mandibular first premolars and molars

References

Andrews LF. The six keys to normal occlusion. Am J Orthod. 1972;62(3):296–309.

Clark JR, Evans RD. Functional occlusion: I. A review. J Orthod. 2001;28(1):76–81.

Miethke RR, Melsen B. Effect of variation in tooth morphology and bracket position on first and third order correction with preadjusted appliances. Am J Orthod Dentofac Orthop. 1999;116(3):329–35.

Owens AM, Johal A. Near-end of treatment panoramic radiograph in the assessment of mesiodistal root angulation. Angle Orthod. 2008;78(3):475–81.

Poling R. A method of finishing the occlusion. Am J Orthod Dentofac Orthop. 1999;115(5):476–87.

Wire Bending

9

Modern fixed appliances are programmed to deliver a desired prescription of tooth movement through a combination of different stages of treatment based on ligation of straight archwires into the bracket slot. Three 'orders' of control of tooth movement are incorporated in the bracket design: first order ('in-out' and rotational control), second order (mesio-distal angulation or 'tip') and third order (inclination or torque) correction. However, in reality the ideal alignment and occlusion are relatively rarely achieved. As such, wire bending is often required to detail the final outcome and is also occasionally required to facilitate achievement of other objectives including overbite reduction and space closure.

Factors which influence tooth positioning during fixed appliance therapy and ultimately the outcome include variation in tooth morphology (Dellinger 1978), errors in relation to bracket placement (Germane et al. 1989), undiagnosed tooth size discrepancies and variations in the underlying skeletal pattern. These can be regarded as patient and operator factors; however, the appliance design itself can also contribute with 'play' in the bracket-archwire system because of oversized bracket slots and undersized archwires precluding the full expression of the bracket prescription (Cash et al. 2004).

Optimal treatment results during the finishing stages of treatment (Chap. 8) are often contingent on localised wire bending to correct individual final tooth position in all three dimensions (antero-posterior, transverse and vertical). Wire bending may be undertaken over 2–3 visits prior to removal of the fixed appliances. The practical steps involvement in correcting common first, second and third order discrepancies as well as facilitating overbite reduction using wire bending are outlined below.

P. Fleming, J. Seehra, *Fixed Orthodontic Appliances*, BDJ Clinician's Guides,
https://doi.org/10.1007/978-3-030-12165-5_9

9.1 Wire Bending: Practical Steps

General wire bending skills require time and practice to perfect. For most bends (with the exception of third order), it is important that the pliers are used to hold or stabilise the wire with the bends made with digital pressure only.

9.2 Wire Bending: Segments

9.2.1 Overbite Reduction: Curve of Spee Variations

Reversed curve of Spee can be added to the mandibular arch to promote extrusion of the premolars with distal tipping of the posterior teeth (see Chap. 6). This configuration promotes overbite reduction and can be introduced with finger pressure producing a maximal depth of curve of approx. 5 mm. Less commonly, similar bends can be introduced in the maxillary wire to assist with overbite reduction but also advancement of maxillary incisors in Class II division 2 cases. Supplementary torque can be added to counteract the likelihood of incisor proclination as required.

9.2.2 Torque Application

Torque bends essentially involve twisting of the arch wire and rely on active bending with pliers (rather than finger pressure). Torque bends can be applied actively to produce new torque (inclination) movement or passively to maintain torque already obtained. Torque prescription is incorporated within the pre-adjusted bracket system, but alteration may be required locally or in a segment for optimal inter- and intra-arch features. Uniform amounts of torque can be placed with continuous torque bends; however, gradation can also be introduced with 'progressive' torque increasing posteriorly in the mandibular arch, in particular.

9.2.3 Space-Closing Loops

With the popularity of sliding mechanics in modern fixed appliance treatment, the use of closing loops appears to be close to obsolete. However, during the finishing stages, closing loops such as Sandusky-type or omega closing loop can be useful adjuncts (Fig. 9.1a, b). They are highly effective at closing residual spaces as they are 'frictionless'. A rectangular stainless steel (0.017 × 0.025 or 0.019 × 0.025 in.) or TMA wire may be used. Additional benefits of using the rectangular wire configuration are torque control or supplementation. Torque can be placed into the incisor region while closing the residual space and maintaining the buccal occlusion (Fig. 9.1c).

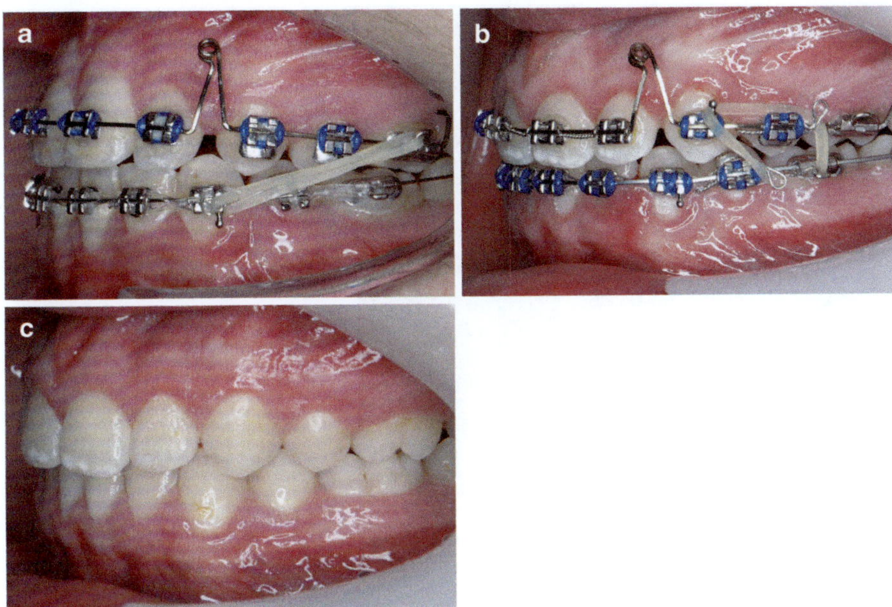

Fig. 9.1 (a–c) A Sandusky closing loop (**a**) in conjunction with Class III traction (**b**) and box elastic (**c**) to facilitate space closure in the maxillary arch and occlusal settling

9.3 Wire Bending: Individual Teeth

9.3.1 In-Out and Rotational Correction (First Order)

Simple buccal offset and inset bends can be made to compensate for differences in the thickness of teeth, bracket bases and cement lutes. Again, these are made in the horizontal plane but involve symmetrical bends. Significant buccal or lingual insets can induce inclination changes with buccal and lingual flaring, respectively.

A formable archwire (round stainless steel or rectangular stainless steel or TMA) can be coordinated to the arch form using the study models as a reference. The wire is cut to length but with limited excess to compensate for the bend. Intra-orally, the contact points between the teeth adjacent to the tooth (e.g. LR3) requiring correction can be marked using a Chinagraph pencil on the archwire (Fig. 9.2a, b).

Using pliers (e.g. light wires) (Chap. 2), the bends are made in the archwire to rotate the crown of the LR3 in the mesio-labial direction (Fig. 9.2c). Before replacing the archwire, it is checked for flatness and arch form (Fig. 9.2d). Positive pressure is required on the first order correction bend to ensure full wire seating. The wire can be held into the bracket slot using finger pressure or a ligature director before ligating the archwire with a positive (figure-of-eight) ormolast or short stainless steel ligature (Fig. 9.2e).

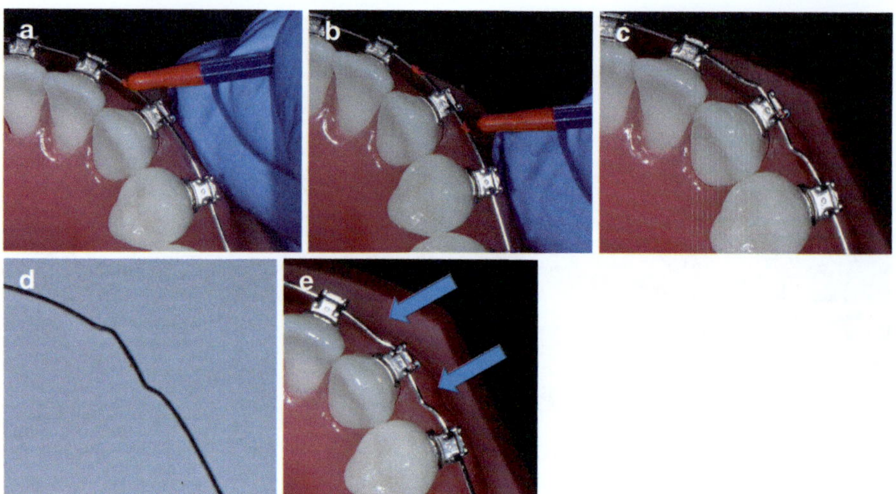

Fig. 9.2 (**a**–**e**) A derotation bend to rotate the mandibular right canine mesio-buccally. A china-graph pencil is useful to guide the location of the bends

9.3.2 Angulation Error Correction (Second Order)

Tip bends can be placed in the archwire to move the root mesially and the crown distally (Fig. 9.3a) or conversely the root distally and the crown mesially (Fig. 9.3b). It is important to ensure the 'peaks' (Fig. 9.3a, b; black arrows) of the bends are in the same horizontal plane as the archwire with no step present to avoid the introduction of vertical changes in the occlusal plane. The archwire (typically round or rectangular stainless steel or TMA) is coordinated and cut to length but with excess to allow for the wire bends. Intra-orally, using a marker, the contact points between the adjacent to the target teeth (e.g. UL1) are marked on the archwire (Fig. 9.3c, d). Using pliers (e.g. light wires) (Chap. 2), the bends are introduced into the archwire to move (tip) the root of the UL1 in a mesial direction and the crown of the UL1 distally (Fig. 9.3d, e). The wire is then inspected to ensure that the plane has otherwise been maintained. It is then ligated in place; the ligation mechanism is less important than is the case for first order bends as the vertical bends ensure that the wire interacts with the gingival and occlusal walls of the slot, rather than the ligature (Fig. 9.3f).

9.3.3 Inclination Error Correction (Third Order)

A rectangular archwire (often 0.019 × 0.025-in. stainless steel or Beta-Titanium) is ideal for torque delivery allowing three-dimensional control. Larger dimension wires (0.021 × 0.025 in.) can be considered although these do increase force levels considerably. A similar process is observed as for first and second order corrections with arch co-ordination.

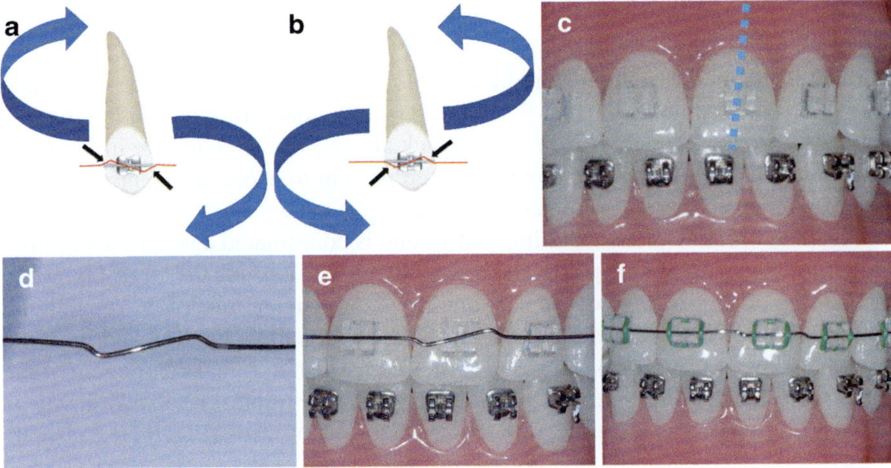

Fig. 9.3 (**a–f**) An angulation (second order) bend to tip the crown of the maxillary left central incisor distally (**b–f**)

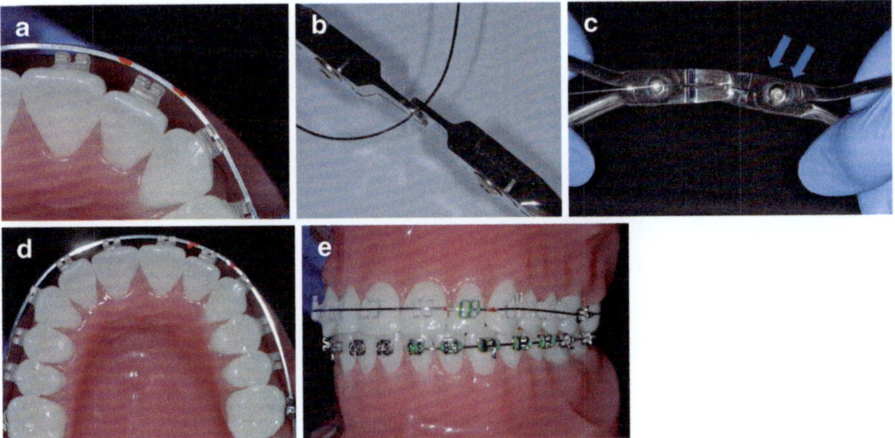

Fig. 9.4 (**a–e**) A torque (second order) placed with Tweeds forceps to torque the root of the maxillary left lateral incisor

For local wire bends torqueing pliers (Tweeds) (Chap. 2) may be used to bend the archwire in the UL2 region only (Fig. 9.4a, b). It can be difficult to determine the direction in which to bend the archwire to introduce the desired correction. As a guide it may be helpful to visualise that the bend that is made in the archwire is the direction you want to move the root of the tooth. For example, labial root torque for the UL2 is being introduced as the pliers in the right hand are moved in a downward direction (Fig. 9.4c). For the archwire to be ligated relatively easily, it is recommended that a third order bend of no more than 12° is placed (Fig. 9.4d). The archwire is then ligated into the bracket slot securely. In order to ensure full expression of the local inclination bend, it is advisable to attempt secure ligation of the neighbouring teeth in order to maximise friction and limit the risk of wire play (Fig. 9.4e).

9.3.4 Vertical Bends

Vertical bends in the archwire can be made to either intrude (Fig. 9.5a) or extrude (Fig. 9.5b) individual teeth (Fig. 9.5c–g). As with second order bends, it is important to ensure the 'slopes' (Fig. 9.5a, b; black arrows) of the bends are in the same horizontal plane as the archwire with no step present to avoid iatrogenic introduction of vertical changes in the occlusal plane.

Again a formable archwire is imperative and is coordinated against the required arch form. Using light wire pliers, the bends are made to extrude the UL4 (Fig. 9.5j). Depending on the stiffness of the wire and the desired magnitude of movement, the height of the vertical bend should not exceed 2 mm to allow ligation and limit the risk of discomfort and bracket debond (Fig. 9.5k). The horizontal component of the archwire bend is ligated into the bracket slot with an ormolast relatively easily as the bend is held in place by the gingival or occlusal slot walls (Fig. 9.5l).

Fig. 9.5 (**c**–**i**). UR1 had previously sustained trauma and had associated recession with discoloration at the gingival margin. As there was a high smile line, a decision was made to replace the pre-existing crown and to attempt extrusion of UR1 to promote a more harmonious gingival architecture. This would necessitate reduction in the height of the existing crown with extrusion (**c**). The attachment height on the UR1 was gauged using the gingival margins as a reference point to allow extrusion in initial NiTi aligning wires (**d**). Thereafter, vertical offset bends were placed in 0.018-inch SS to promote further gradual extrusion (**e**–**f**) promoting improvement in the gingival aesthetics (**g**) prior to definitive restoration. A permanent crown with improved aesthetics and gingival harmony was subsequently placed (**h**, **i**)

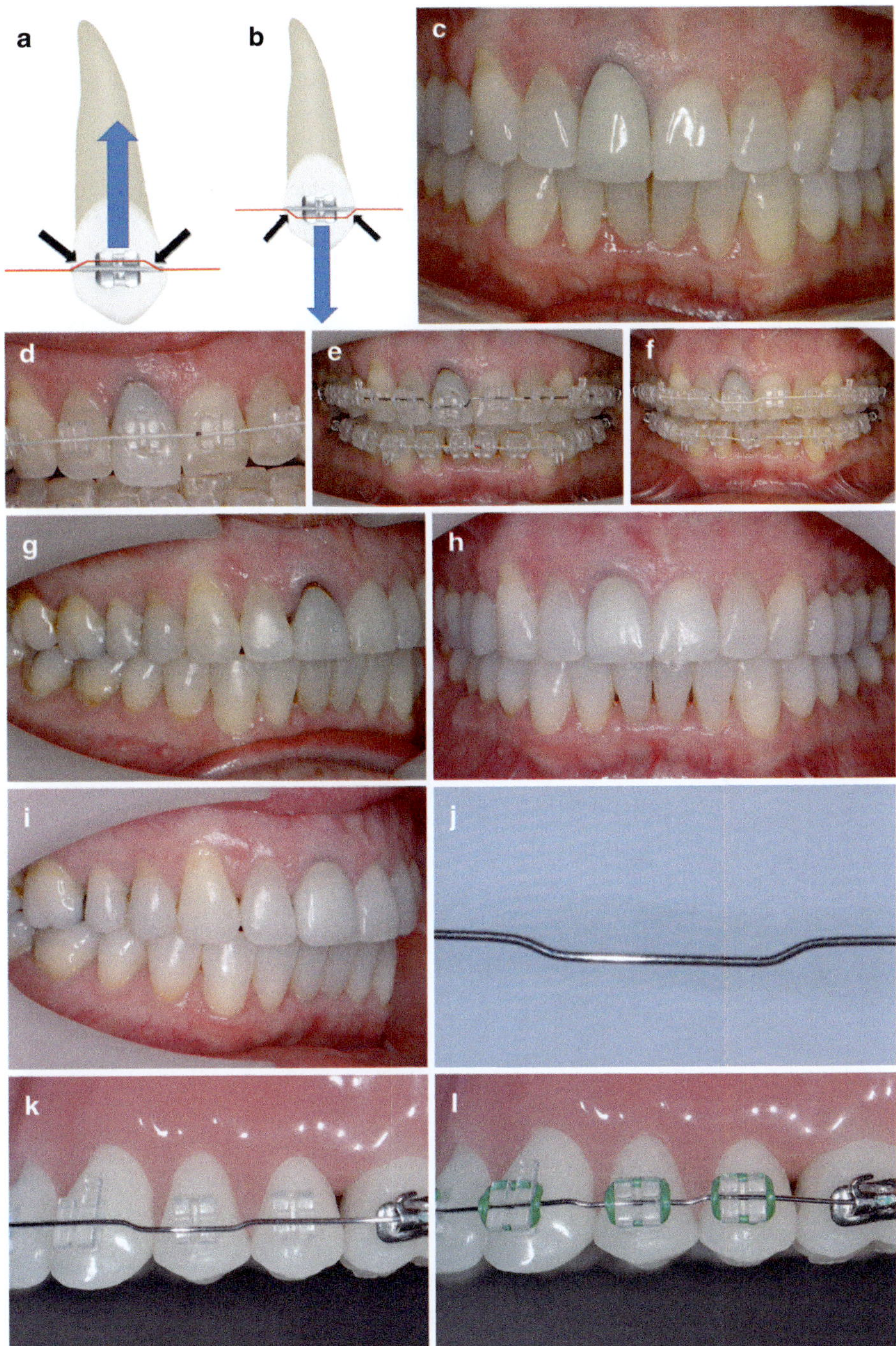
a
b
c
d
e
f
g
h
i
j
k
l

References

Cash AC, Good SA, Curtis RV, McDonald F. An evaluation of slot size in orthodontic brackets—are standards as expected? Angle Orthod. 2004;74(4):450–3.

Dellinger EL. A scientific assessment of the straight-wire appliance. Am J Orthod. 1978;73(3):290–9.

Germane N, Bentley BE Jr, Isaacson RJ. Three biologic variables modifying faciolingual tooth angulation by straight-wire appliances. Am J Orthod Dentofac Orthop. 1989;96(4):312–9.

Removal of Fixed Appliances

10

The technique for removing fixed appliances is well-established and typically involves the following steps: debonding of fixed appliance attachments, removal of adhesive remnants from the tooth surface using a tungsten carbide bur and polishing of the enamel surface (Retief and Denys 1979). Enamel loss following the removal of composite residue is commonplace (Ryf et al. 2012). Therefore, various alternatives to burs have been proposed including hand instruments, stones, wheels and discs, scalers, lasers and pumice or zirconium paste. Surface changes reduce the resistance of enamel to bacterial and organic acid attack increasing susceptibility to demineralisation and dental caries.

The critical threshold value of enamel surface roughness for bacterial adhesion has been established at 0.2 μm (Bollen et al. 1997). However, conventional methods of adhesive removal, including scalers and dental burs, may lead to visible surface roughness with grooves ranging from 10 to 20 μm deep and loss of up to 100 μm thickness of enamel (Dumore and Fried 2000).

The development of enamel microcracks may also predispose the tooth to both further loss of enamel structure and dental caries secondary to bacterial colonisation. The number of microcracks is likely to increase following fixed appliance removal (Dumbryte et al. 2018). Consequently, it is important that every precaution is undertaken to ensure the integrity of the enamel surface is maintained as much as possible when debonding fixed appliances. The practical steps involved in the removal of fixed appliances are outlined below.

P. Fleming, J. Seehra, *Fixed Orthodontic Appliances*, BDJ Clinician's Guides,
https://doi.org/10.1007/978-3-030-12165-5_10

Box 10.1 Removing Fixed Attachments from Restored Teeth

When fixed appliance attachments have been bonded to heavily-restored teeth or indirect restorations, extra care should be taken as restorations or unsupported enamel may be prone to fracture and indirect restorations can be inadvertently loosened and require replacement or recementation. In addition, heavily-restored teeth may predispose the remaining tooth surface to fracture of the enamel surface during the removal of attachments (Fig. 10.1a, b). Diligent removal of all excess adhesive is sensible prior to attempting debond in susceptible teeth.

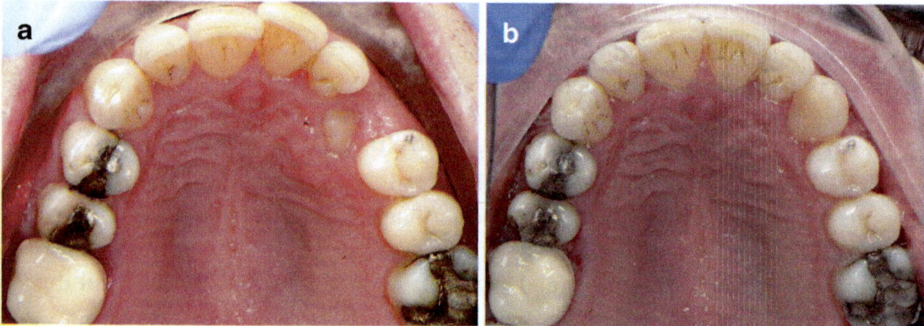

Fig. 10.1 (**a**, **b**) Following orthodontic alignment of the UL3 in an adult with a restored dentition (**a**), fracture of the distal aspect of the buccal surface of the restored UR5 occurred during the removal of the fixed appliance (**b**)

Box 10.2 Removal of Ceramic Brackets

The bond strength of ceramic brackets bonded to the enamel surface compared to stainless steel brackets is considerably higher (Joseph and Rossouw 1990). Clinically, this may be beneficial in avoiding unscheduled breakages of fixed appliance attachments during treatment. However, this may pose a problem when removing ceramic attachments as the risk of enamel surface damage is increased (Joseph and Rossouw 1990). It is advised to follow tailored manufacturer's instructions when removing ceramic fixed appliances. This may involve modifying the debonding technique by removing the archwire initially along with excess composite flash around brackets. Bespoke ceramic bracket debonding pliers are also produced to simplify attachment removal in a number of ceramic systems (Fig. 10.2a–c).

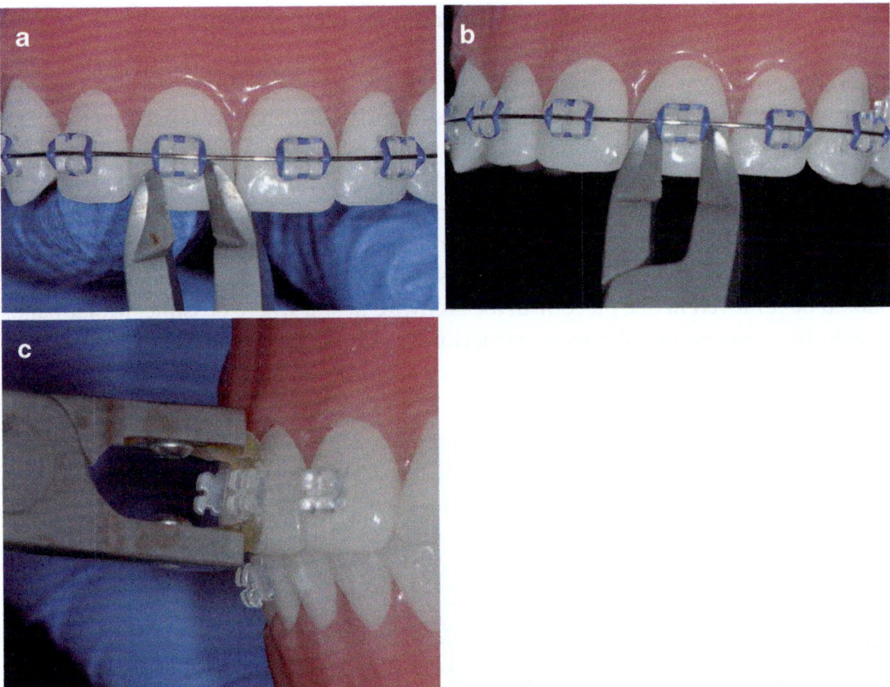

Fig. 10.2 (**a–c**) Bespoke pliers may be used to remove ceramic attachments

Box 10.3 Alternative Approaches for Adhesive Removal

Adhesive removal with tungsten carbide burs has been linked to more enamel roughness compared to other burs, or white stones using a range of in vitro assessment techniques. Laboratory techniques (e.g. profilometry) have illustrated that the use of tungsten carbide burs increases enamel surface roughness regardless of the type of adhesive used. Propulsion of bioactive glasses has shown promise in relation to adhesive removal (Banerjee et al. 2008; Taha et al. 2018) in laboratory-based studies. These do also offer the potential advantage of enamel remineralisation related to phosphate and fluoride content. Effective adhesive removal, however, involves a trade-off between efficiency and safety with larger, more irregular and coarser particles likely to produce more rapid removal but risking more enamel damage. As such, further material refinement is required in order to improve physical and handling properties.

10.1 Removal of Fixed Appliances: Practical Steps

Prior to the removal of the fixed appliance, the appliance should be inspected for any missing modules, loose or lost attachments (Fig. 10.3a). The most distal attachment, commonly a molar tube or band, can be secured by cinching the distal aspect of the archwire (Fig. 10.3b) to prevent this from sliding off the terminal end of the wire with associated risk of ingestion or inhalation. In addition, a separator can be placed on the molar hook gripping the end of the archwire using mosquito forceps (Fig. 10.3c–f).

To simplify removal and prevent the loss of individual attachments, the appliance should be removed in one piece with the archwire in situ where possible. Molar bands should be loosened initially using posterior band remover pliers. For the removal of maxillary molar bands, bands are loosened from the palatal aspect initially as the

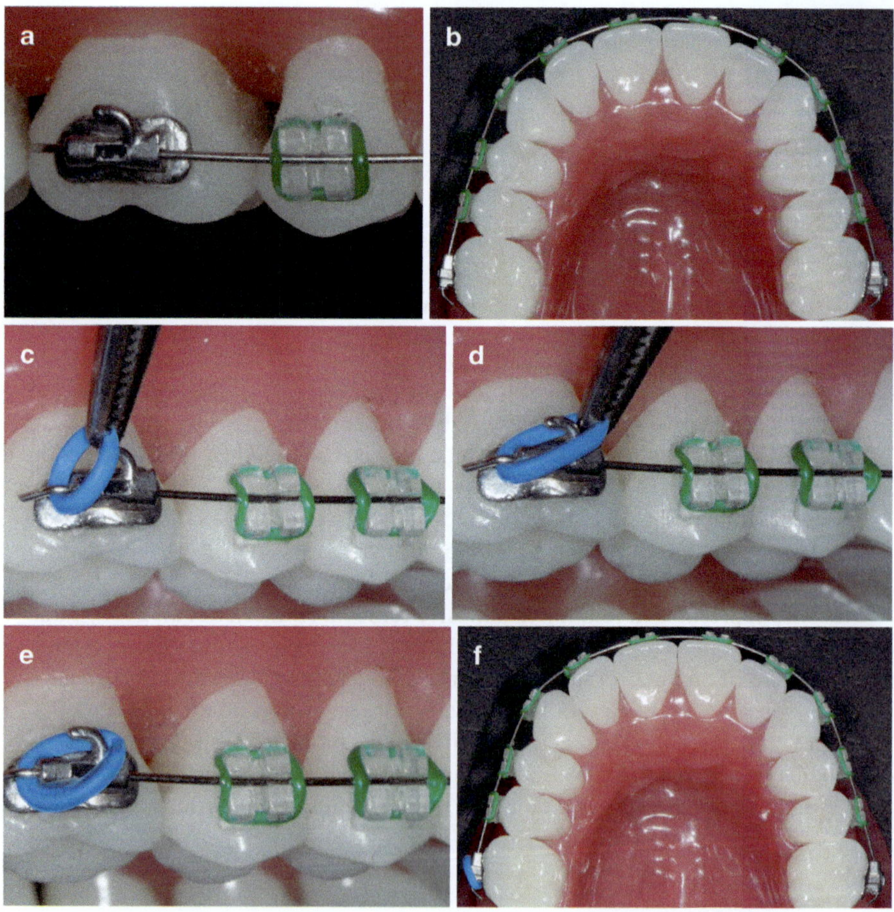

Fig. 10.3 (**a–f**) Ideally, the fixed appliance should be removed en masse. The distal ends can be cinched (**b**) or elastomeric modules placed around the terminal molar attachments to prevent dislodgement (and possible ingestion) of the terminal attachments during debonding

palatal surface does not normally present an undercut. The gingival edge of the band on the palatal surface should be engaged with the beak of the posterior band remover pliers, while the rubber stop rests on the occlusal surface of the tooth. The band is then gently lifted away from the tooth surface (Fig. 10.4a–h). For mandibular molar bands, the posterior band remover pliers should engage the gingival edge of the band from the buccal aspect with the rubber stop resting on the occlusal surface (Fig. 10.4i–l).

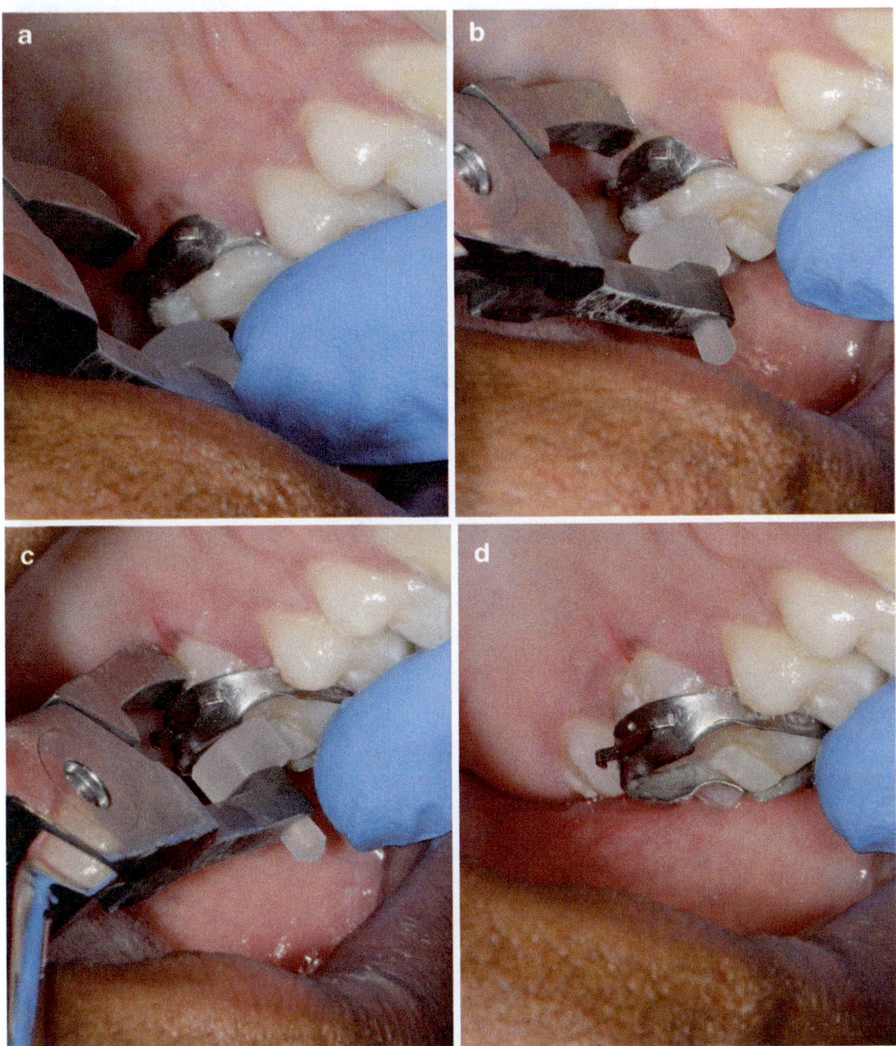

Fig. 10.4 (**a–l**) Removal of molar bands using posterior band remover pliers

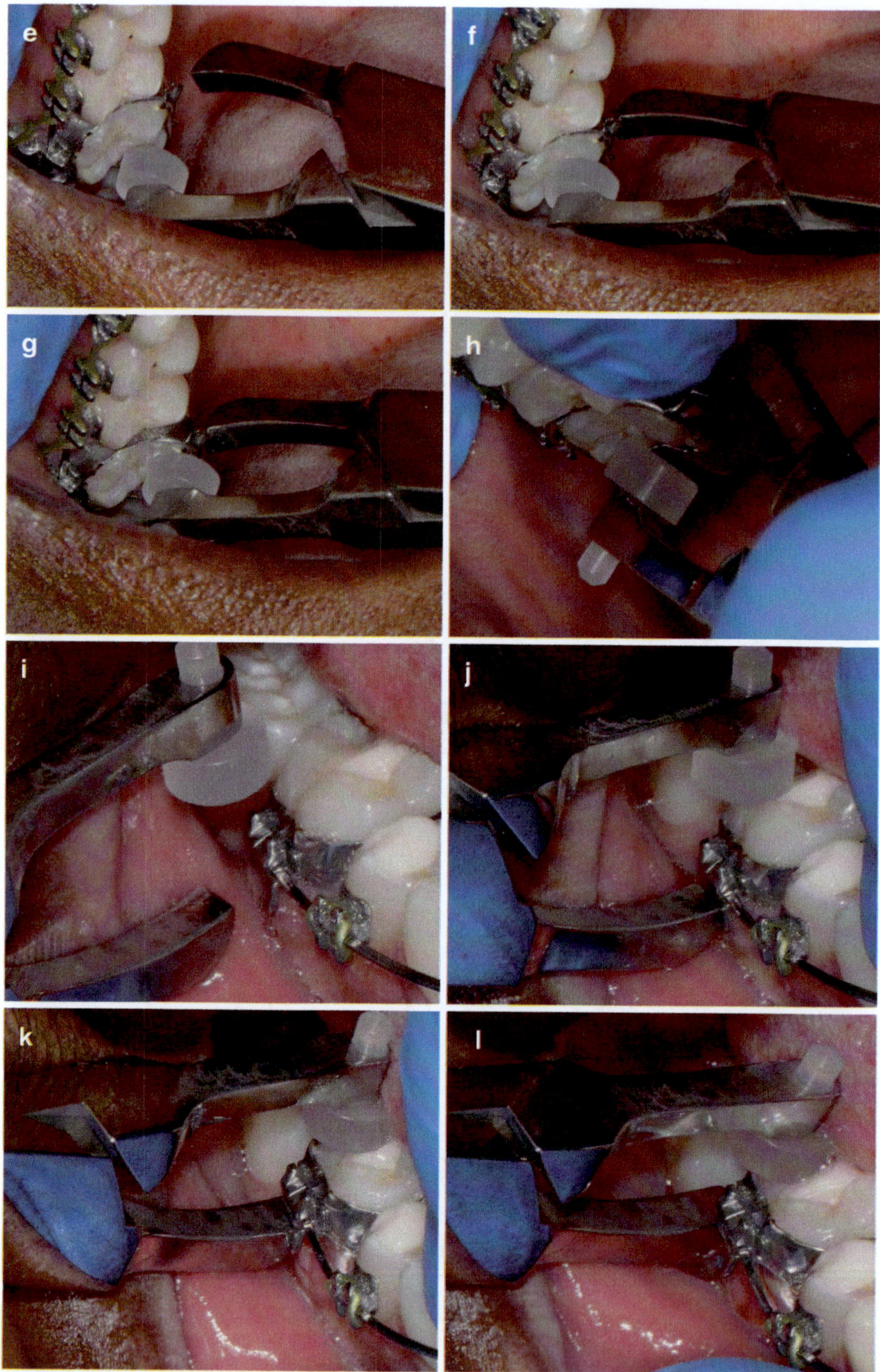

Fig. 10.4 (continued)

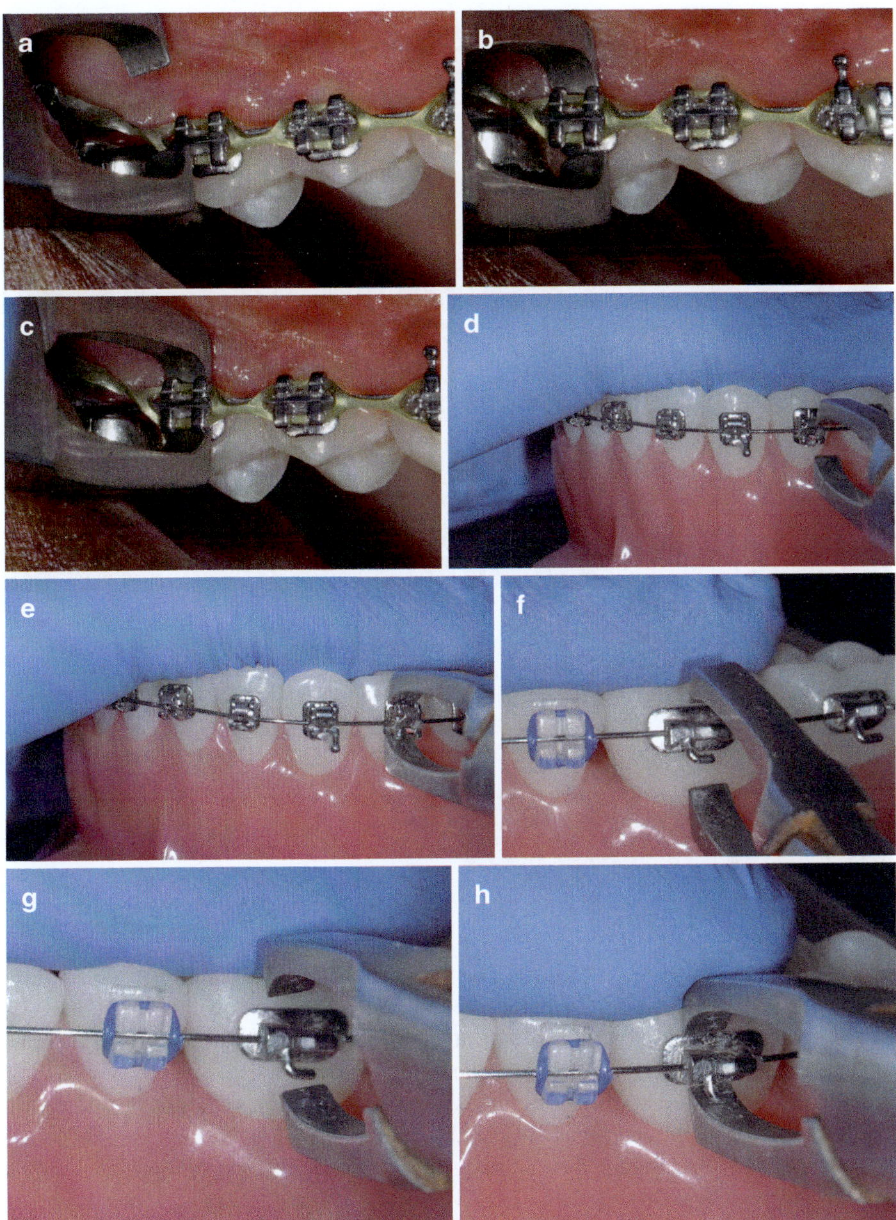

Fig. 10.5 (**a–m**) Removal of fixed appliances en masse with gentle pressure involving a debond pliers (**a–h**) and a band remover (**i–m**), as required

When removing molar tubes or brackets, the tips of the bracket remover pliers should be engaged around the gingival and occlusal aspects (Fig. 10.5a–c). Very gentle pressure is applied while supporting the tooth with finger pressure to squeeze the bracket, ideally inducing a bond failure between the bracket base and surface

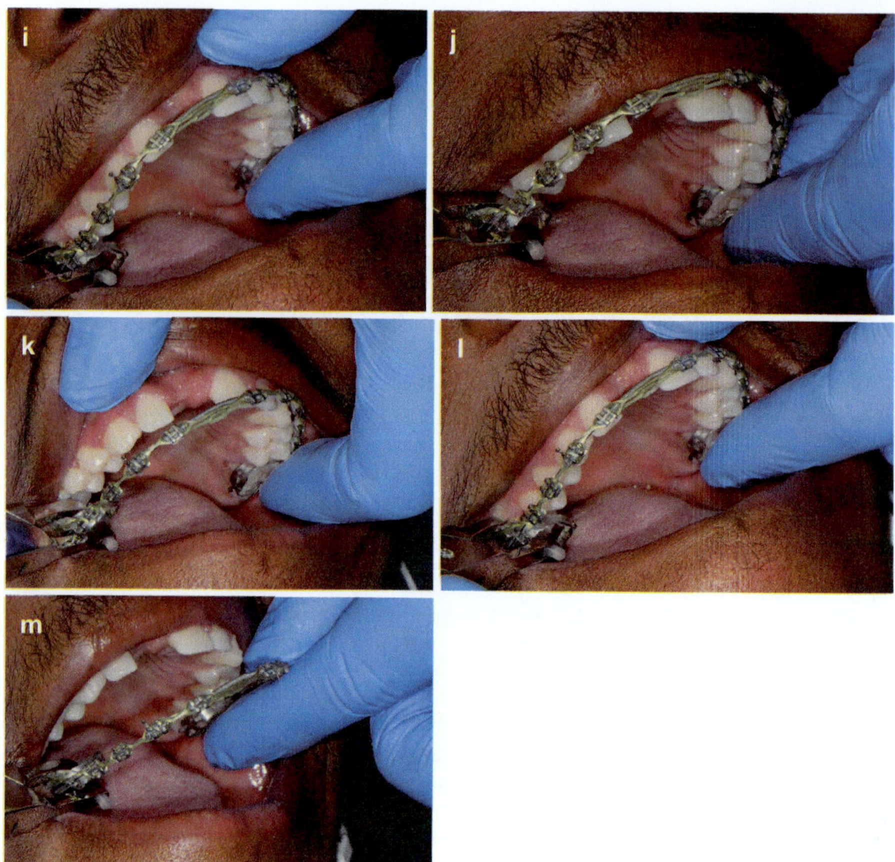

Fig. 10.5 (continued)

layer of composite (Fig. 10.5d–h). The tooth itself can be stabilised with gentle finger pressure or by asking the patient to bite on cotton roll or wax to limit discomfort during bracket removal. Once all attachments have been debonded, the appliance is held securely and removed in one piece (Fig. 10.5i–m).

The most accepted approach to adhesive removal remains the use of a tungsten carbide bur in a slow handpiece (Fig. 10.6a). The bur should be held parallel to the tooth surface while moving it in a brush fashion to remove the composite, while a secure finger rest is maintained (Fig. 10.6b–g). During composite removal, the flutes of the bur can become occluded with composite fragments resulting in reduced efficiency, an increase in frictional forces and generation of heat which can be conducted to the soft tissues via the metallic handpiece. To avoid the risk of iatrogenic damage, the soft tissues should be retracted fully during the removal of the fixed appliance (Fig. 10.6h).

A high-volume suction aspirator should be held near the tooth surface to collect the dust particles or fragments during the removal of the composite (Fig. 10.6i, j).

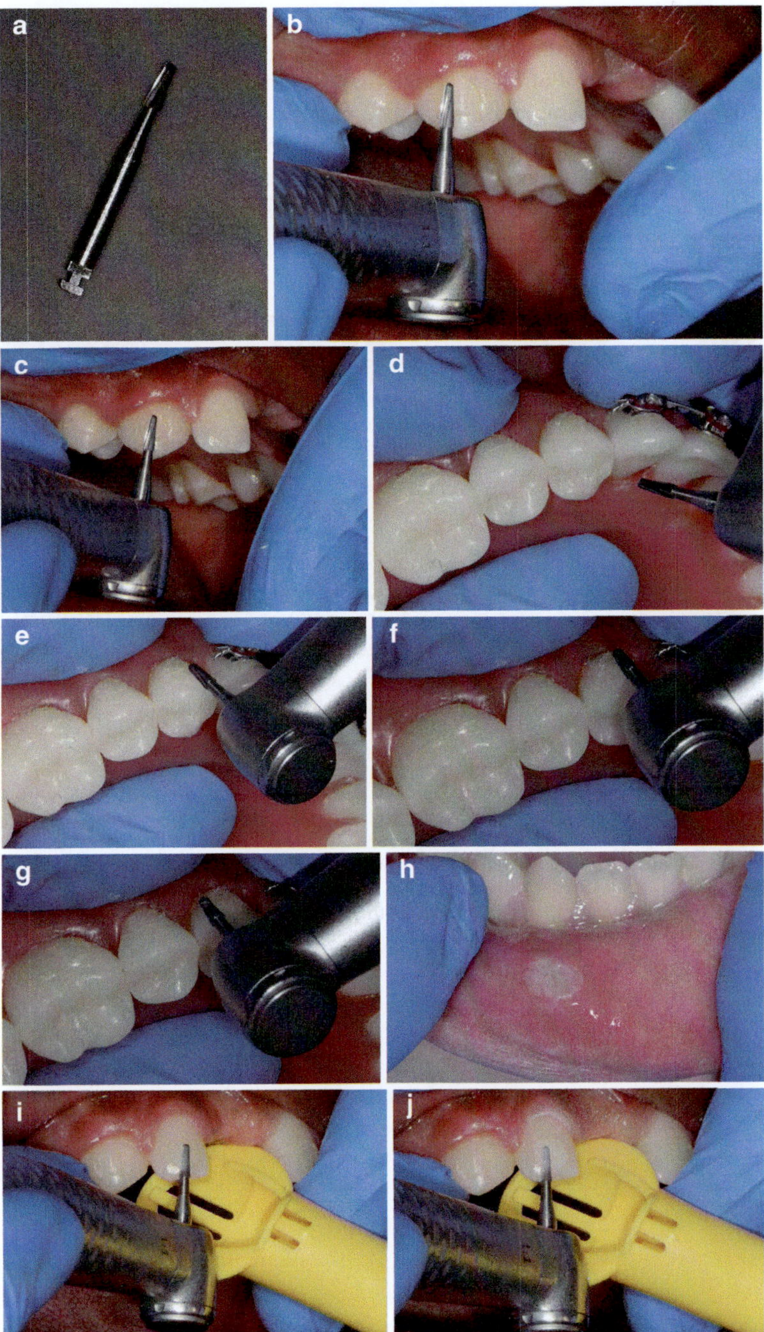

Fig. 10.6 (**a**–**j**) Removal of adhesive material using tungsten carbide burs (**a**–**j**). Care should be taken to avoid overheating with traumatic ulceration of the lower lip as a result of contact with a slow handpiece during the removal of an upper fixed appliance 1 week earlier (**h**)

Composite resin adhesive tends to assume a noticeably whiter appearance during debonding. Once this white appearance diminishes, it likely indicates that all adhesive has been removed. Following the removal of the composite, the surface of the tooth can be polished using non-fluoridated pumice paste for approximately 20 seconds per tooth and the surface inspected for any residual adhesive remnants (Fig. 10.7a–d). Polishing, however, has little effect on enamel surface roughness values with no tangible effect on the grooves or pits induced during enamel clean-up (Gwinnett and Gorelick 1977).

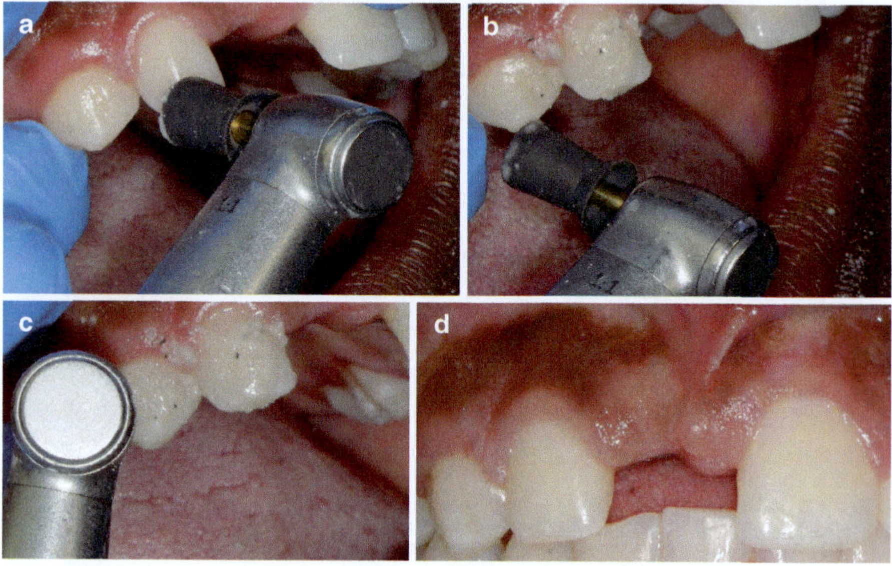

Fig. 10.7 (**a**–**d**) The enamel surface of the tooth can be polished using non-fluoridated pumice paste for 20 seconds per tooth

References

Banerjee A, Paolinelis G, Socker M, McDonald F, Watson TF. An in vitro investigation of the effectiveness of bioactive glass air-abrasion in the 'selective' removal of orthodontic resin adhesive. Eur J Oral Sci. 2008;116(5):488–92.

Bollen CM, Lambrechts P, Quirynen M. Comparison of surface roughness of oral hard materials to the threshold surface roughness for bacterial plaque retention: a review of the literature. Dent Mater. 1997;13(4):258–69.

Dumbryte I, Vebriene J, Linkeviciene L, Malinauskas M. Enamel microcracks in the form of tooth damage during orthodontic debonding: a systematic review and meta-analysis of in vitro studies. Eur J Orthod. 2018;40:636.

Dumore T, Fried D. Selective ablation of orthodontic composite by using sub-microsecond IR laser pulses with optical feedback. Lasers Surg Med. 2000;27(2):103–10.

Gwinnett AJ, Gorelick L. Microscopic evaluation of enamel after debonding: clinical application. Am J Orthod. 1977;71(6):651–65.

Joseph VP, Rossouw E. The shear bond strengths of stainless steel and ceramic brackets used with chemically and light-activated composite resins. Am J Orthod Dentofac Orthop. 1990;97(2):121–5.

Retief DH, Denys FR. Finishing of enamel surfaces after debonding of orthodontic attachments. Angle Orthod. 1979;49(1):1–10.

Ryf S, Flury S, Palaniappan S, Lussi A, van Meerbeek B, Zimmerli B. Enamel loss and adhesive remnants following bracket removal and various clean-up procedures in vitro. Eur J Orthod. 2012;34(1):25–32.

Taha AA, Hill RG, Fleming PS, Patel MP. Development of a novel bioactive glass for air-abrasion to selectively remove orthodontic adhesives. Clin Oral Investig. 2018;22(4):1839–49.

11 Orthodontic Retention

The use of retainers in orthodontics is an accepted and integral phase of treatment. The necessity for retention following comprehensive treatment cannot be disputed and indeed was alluded to by orthodontic pioneers many of whom advocated prolonged or even lifelong retention (Case 2003).

The rationale for retention is threefold mitigating against:

- Unstable tooth positioning: A range of orthodontic tooth movements are known to be particularly susceptible to relapse. These include advancement of the mandibular incisors and mandibular inter-canine width expansion.
- Physiological recovery: Physiological recovery of the alveolus, periodontal ligament and particularly the supracrestal fibres is gradual with more than 6 months believed to be required for this process to occur. Retainers are therefore considered indispensable over this period as a minimum.
- Growth and maturational change: Characteristic changes affect the dentition with lower anterior irregularity, in particular, known to increase over time for a variety of reasons (Sinclair and Little 1983). As such, indefinite retention is a prerequisite if optimal intra-arch alignment, in particular, is to be preserved.

Removable retainers offer a relatively simple approach to maintaining treated results but do place an onus on compliance, particularly in the long term. Removable retainers may be provided in isolation or may complement fixed retention in view of potential tooth movement posteriorly and indeed anterior change related to fixed retainer failure or activation.

Research concerning the relative merits of fixed and removable retention protocols has given slightly conflicting results with a 12-month follow-up (Edman Tynelius et al. 2010) finding no meaningful difference in relapse found between three groups with a vacuum-formed retainer in the maxilla and bonded canine-to-canine retainer in the mandible, Essix-type retainer in the maxilla combined with stripping of lower anterior interproximal surfaces, or a positioner in both arches.

P. Fleming, J. Seehra, *Fixed Orthodontic Appliances*, BDJ Clinician's Guides,
https://doi.org/10.1007/978-3-030-12165-5_11

A more recent study carried out in the UK has alluded to superiority of fixed retention over removable alternatives in a longer-term (4-year) follow-up. This difference stems from waning levels of compliance with removable retention over time with just 33% wearing retainers diligently over 2 years following completion of active treatment (Al-Moghrabi et al. 2018). It is likely, therefore, that fixed approaches may offer a more credible prospect of indefinite correction following orthodontics.

Box 11.1 Which Removable Retainer Is Most Effective?

Hawley, Begg and Essix-type retainers are amongst the most popular removable retainers. A number of randomised controlled trials have considered the relative benefits of these retainers both with respect to objective and subjective measures. Begg retainers are now rarely used. They do offer the potential for unimpeded occlusal settling with absence of acrylic coverage or posterior clasping; however, they may offer less control of tooth movement than more accepted alternatives. Essix-type retainers are generally well-tolerated and have good aesthetics (Fig. 11.1a). They do, however, tend to impede posterior occlusal settling post-treatment, may lack sufficient rigidity to maintain transverse expansion and are prone to fracture and distortion, although thicker forms may mitigate against these issues. Conversely, Hawley retainers are more durable and more rigid, thereby facilitating maintenance of expansion while also lacking occlusal coverage and therefore assisting in settling the posterior occlusion (Fig. 11.1b, c). They are, however, less aesthetic and therefore less well-tolerated. Comparative research has suggested that Essix retainers are preferable to Hawley with respect to compliance, tolerance and cost-efficacy in the short term (Hichens et al. 2007; Rowland et al. 2007).

In terms of international use, a survey in the USA has highlighted a preference for maxillary Hawley retainers (58%) and mandibular fixed lingual retainers with full-time wear of removable retainers advocated for less than 9 months (Valiathan and Hughes 2010), although a preference for vacuum-formed retainers was identified in a more recent American study (Pratt et al. 2011). Similar findings were revealed in a survey in the UK, with vacuum-formed retainers also generally preferred to Hawley retainers (Singh et al. 2009).

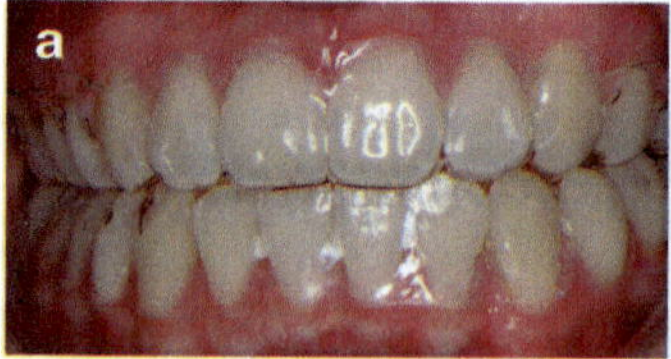

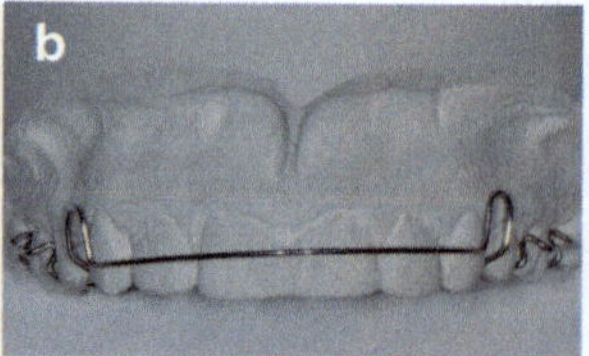

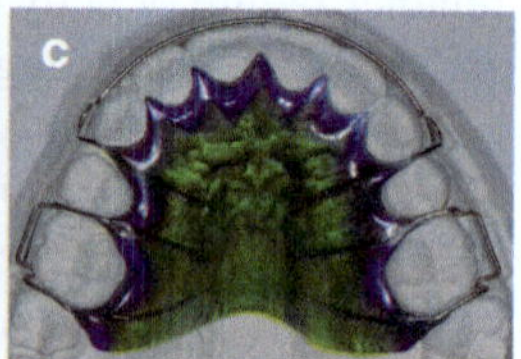

Fig. 11.1 (**a**–**c**) Essix-type retainers (**a**) and maxillary arch Hawley retainer (**b**, **c**)

A large randomised trial in the UK involving 397 patients compared both objective (Rowland et al. 2007) and economic and subjective considerations (Hichens et al. 2007) over a 6-month retention period in a single practice. Greater irregularity was observed in the anterior region with Hawley than with Essix-type retainers, with slightly more pronounced differences in the mandibular (0.56 mm) than the maxillary (0.25 mm) anterior region. In addition, Essix-type retainers were found to be more cost-effective than Hawley retainers with patients also preferring Essix-type retainers.

A further issue with removable retainers is longevity. A randomised study based in China attempted to address this question by considering survival time with Essix and Hawley retainers, although the follow-up period was limited to 12 months (Sun et al. 2011). Of 120 adolescent patients with dual-arch retention, 34 Hawley and 44 Essix-type retainers fractured. No statistical difference was found with respect to fracture, loss or deterioration of fit. The authors concluded that breakage rates may not influence the choice of retainer; however, this conclusion may not apply with longer periods of retention with some evidence that Hawley retainers may be more durable.

A helpful form of post-treatment change during the retention phase is occlusal settling. In a prospective study with alternate assignment, Sauget et al. (1997) compared the increase in the number of occlusal contacts with either a Hawley retainer worn full-time or an Essix-type retainer on a nights-only basis. The Hawley retainer allowed significantly more settling with a mean difference of 6.5 contacts. The analysis, however, was restricted to a 3-month period.

Box 11.2 Which Design and Material Is Proven Most Effective for Fixed Retainers?

Since their introduction, small-diameter braided or coaxial round stainless steel wires bonded to all mandibular anterior teeth have become established as a gold standard (Fig. 11.2a–f). Prolonged follow-ups have alluded to relatively high failure rates of fixed retainers (Booth et al. 2008) and the propensity for periodontal compromise (Pandis et al. 2007). More recently, alternatives including fibre-reinforced materials and alumina ceramic retainers have been introduced.

Årtun et al. (1997) in a 3-year follow-up compared 0.032-in. plain or spiral canine-and-canine retainers and 0.0205-in. spiral canine-to-canine retainers with a removable retainer. While irregularity increased significantly over the

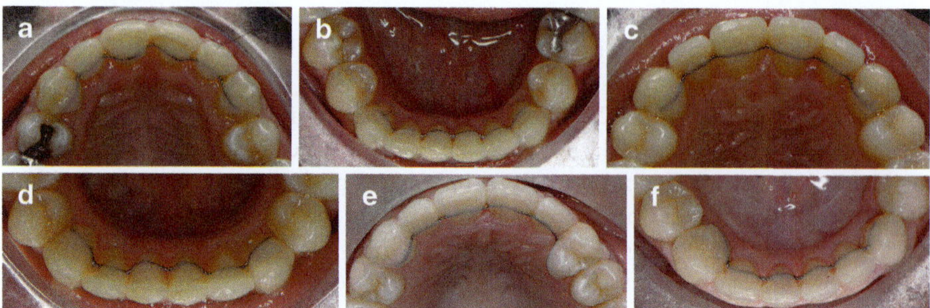

Fig. 11.2 (**a–f**) 0.0175- and 0.0195-in. TwistFlex bonded wires. These can be lab-made and bonded indirectly or bent up at chairside and placed directly. These are in common usage. A potential problem with these may reside in the inherent rigidity in the wire with residual activation or indeed de novo activation due to function leading to force propagation and displacement of terminal teeth over time. Passive placement of the retainer wire is imperative. Indirect placement using transfer jigs may assist with this. Alternatively, use of orthodontic elastics can facilitate placement suspending the wire in place prior to curing of adhesive material

follow-up period, no difference in changes was observed between the respective groups. Störmann and Ehmer (2002) compared customised canine-to-canine retainers (attached to six teeth) with wire diameters of 0.0215" or 0.0195" and a prefabricated canine-and-canine retainer (bonded to two teeth) in respect of detachment rate, relapse, periodontal and oral hygiene problems, as well as subjective patient discomfort. The risk of detachment was significantly lower with canine-and-canine retainers (18%) compared to the 0.0195" canine-to-canine retainer (29%), although the 0.0215" canine-to-canine retainer had the highest detachment risk (53%). Overall, stability was acceptable with both canine-to-canine retainers, while relapse of incisors not bonded to canine-and-canine retainers was common.

Tacken et al. (2010) undertook a comparison between glass fibre-reinforced retainers with one of two fibre compositions and multistrand stainless steel orthodontic retainers in terms of success rate and periodontal implications over a 2-year period. Excessive failure rates were found with glass fibre retainers (51%), while only 12% of the SSW retainers failed. Fracture of upper retainers was observed in 77% of failures, while detachment of lower retainers was common; however, only three lower multistrand steel retainers fractured. Modified gingival index scores also increased more significantly with glass fibre retainers leading the authors to conclude that they should not be recommended for routine use. These conclusions were supported in a more recent uncontrolled prospective follow-up. Ardeshna (2011) reported poor survival rates with fibre-reinforced plastic fixed retainers with a median survival time of just 7.6 months; only 33% survived after 12 months.

Box 11.3 Are Auxiliary Procedures (e.g., Interproximal Reduction or Surgical Adjuncts) of Value or Perhaps More Effective than Use of Retainers?

With the exception of the study by Edman Tynelius et al. (2010) who compared the use of interproximal reduction with other retention protocols, there has been no RCT addressing this question. However, two prospective studies (Taner et al. 2000; Edwards 1988) have considered the relationship between circumferential supracrestal fiberotomy and relapse in conjunction with removable retainer wear. Taner et al. (2000) reported a 2 mm decrease in relapse over a 12-month follow-up period without any attendant periodontal compromise. The study by Edwards (1988) was confounded by a large number of drop-outs and inconsistent duration of removable retainer wear. As such, there remains little evidence to support the use of surgical adjunctive procedures in minimising post-treatment change.

Box 11.4 Should Removable Retainers Be Worn on a Part-Time or Full-Time Basis?

Retention protocols tend to be tailored to individual patients and tend to be governed by operator preference. However, removable retention remains a mainstay of retention. The relative merits of part-time and full-time wear of removable retainers have been evaluated in clinical research, producing very consistent findings.

Based on an analysis of 60 participants, Gill et al. (2007) concluded that there is little difference in lower labial segment stability with either full-time or nights-only wear of Essix-type retainers over a 12-month period (Gill et al. 2007). A further analysis involving Essix retainers confirmed these findings with full-time wear over a 12-month period resulting in little discernible difference in stability compared to part-time wear (Thicket and Power 2010). Similarly, in a 12-month follow-up, Shawesh et al. (2010) noted little difference in irregularity following more prolonged retention with analogous levels of irregularity and crowding following 12 months of full-time wear and 6 months of full-time and 6 months of nights-only wear.

On the basis of these studies, it can be deduced that nights-only wear may be sufficient. This approach also reduces the burden of retention wear and may improve the longevity of retainers, by reducing wear-induced degradation and limiting the potential for loss, improving their cost-effectiveness. As such, full-time wear for a short period (up to 1 week) can be recommended in the first instance before graduating to nights-only retainer wear as this protocol allows for initial adaptation to the retainer while also promoting adequate longevity.

Box 11.5 What Are the Short- and Long-Term Effects of Removable and Fixed Retainers on the Dentition and Supporting Structures?

Long-term retention has generally been accepted to be compatible with periodontal health, although increased plaque and calculus accumulation are likely. Fixed retainers do increase the potential for plaque stagnation with associated risk of periodontal damage; as such, instruction in relation to hygiene measures including use of interproximal brushes and modified dental floss is important (Chap. 12). Booth et al. (2008) in a retrospective cohort study showed no adverse effects of fixed retention on periodontal and gingival health with canine-and-canine retainers. Nevertheless, it would appear sensible to avoid indiscriminate use of lingual fixed retainers particularly in those patients with inadequate oral hygiene.

Pandis et al. (2007) in a retrospective cohort study compared groups having fixed retainers over a prolonged period (9–11 years) and those with relatively short retention periods of up to 6 months. More calculus accumulation, marginal gingival recession and probing depths were noted in the groups with prolonged retention. However, no differences were noted for plaque and gingival indices and bone levels. Similarly, Levin et al. (2008) in an analysis of 92 consecutive subjects reported more lingual gingival recession in association with fixed retainers. Plaque and gingival indices and bleeding on probing were also higher in the presence of fixed retainers.

Prolonged follow-up of subjects with bonded flexible-spiral wires to lower anteriors has been associated with two distinct complications. In particular, Katsaros et al. (2007) have alluded to the development of significant de novo torque differential between adjacent mandibular incisors and buccal inclination and movement of one mandibular canine in isolation. The authors suggest that these unexpected changes may necessitate retreatment with ten patients in whom retainers remained intact found to require further orthodontic correction for these reasons. Apparently, residual stress in the materials may be expressed over time which renders the notion of passive retainers questionable (Fig. 11.3a–c). Clinicians should consider this possibility when planning retention strategies. Recently, stainless steel and 14-carat gold

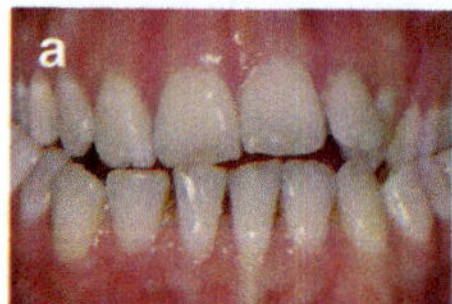

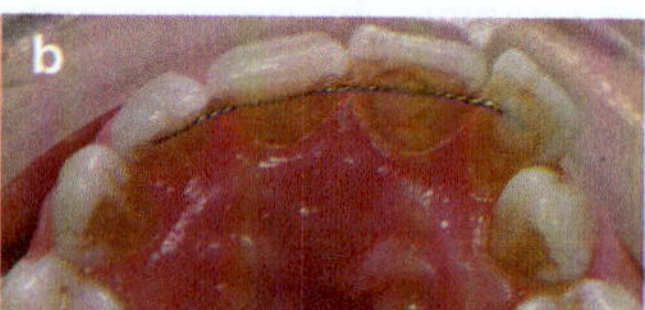

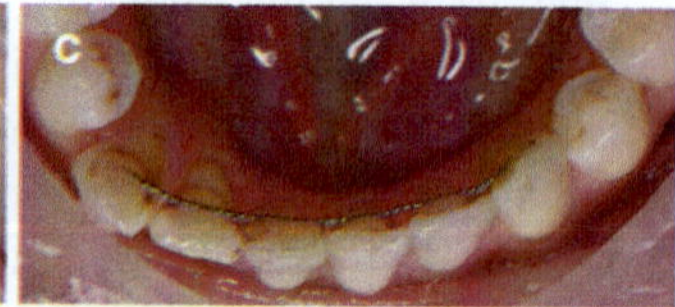

Fig. 11.3 (**a–c**) Post-treatment change arising 10 years following orthodontic treatment with activation of TwistFlex wires leading to marked proclination of UL2 and LR3 with space opening in the lower right quadrant

retainer chains have been introduced which appear passive (Figs. 11.4a–f and 11.5a–h) and do not require pressure to adapt to the tooth; however, at this point there is no evidence in terms of long-term performance or attendant tooth movements.

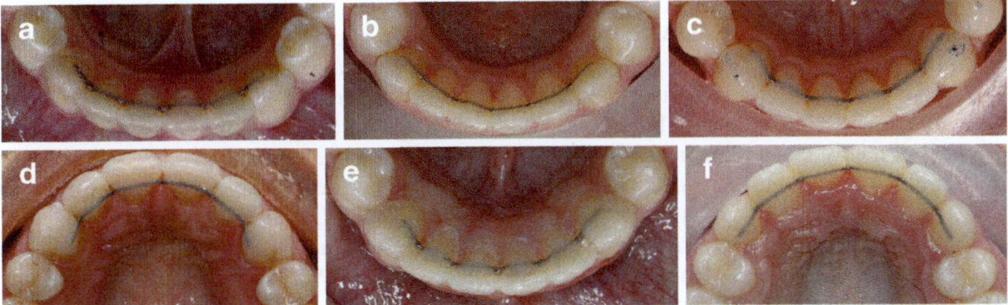

Fig. 11.4 (**a**–**f**) FlexTech bonded wires (14-carat gold and stainless steel variants) bonded from canine to canine with wide coverage of the lingual surfaces and low composite profile

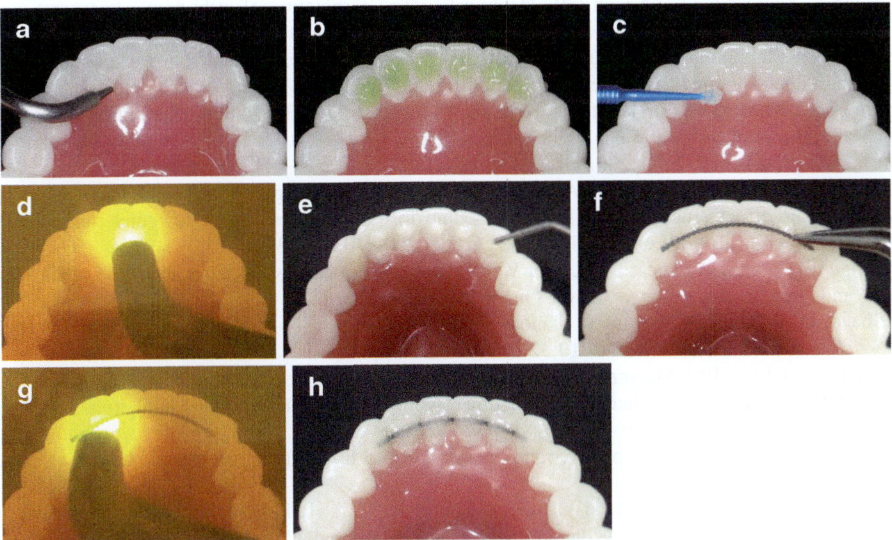

Fig. 11.5 (**a**–**h**) Technique for placing FlexTech bonded retainer wires (courtesy of Mrs. Anna Blazewska-Amin) involving sandblasting of the enamel surface prior to etching and bonding (**a**–**c**). The bonding agent is subsequently light-cured before a small amount of flowable composite is placed centrally on the lingual surfaces (**d**, **e**). The wire is then introduced with a tweezers using the flowable composite to gently tack the wire into position (**f**). The composite it subsequently cured (**g**) before a layer of heavily filled composite is applied (**h**). The latter may be moulded with a small brush and probe aiming to cover a wide surface area but maintaining a relatively thin section. This pattern may enhance comfort by reducing the intrusiveness of the wire while promoting improved bond strength by virtue of the wide coverage

References

Al-Moghrabi D, Johal A, O'Rourke N, Donos N, Pandis N, Gonzales-Marin C, Fleming PS. Effects of fixed vs removable orthodontic retainers on stability and periodontal health: 4-year follow-up of a randomized controlled trial. Am J Orthod Dentofac Orthop. 2018;154(2):167–74.

Ardeshna AP. Clinical evaluation of fiber-reinforced-plastic bonded orthodontic retainers. Am J Orthod Dentofacial Orthop. 2011;139:761–7.

Årtun J, Spadafora AT, Shapiro PA. A 3-year follow-up of various types of orthodontic canine-to-canine retainers. Eur J Orthod. 1997;19:501–9.

Booth FA, Edelman JM, Proffit WR. Twenty-year follow-up of patients with permanently bonded mandibular canine-to-canine retainers. Am J Orthod Dentofac Orthop. 2008;133:70–6.

Case CS. Principles of retention in orthodontia. Am J Orthod Dentofac Orthop. 2003;124:352–61.

Edman Tynelius G, Bondemark L, Lilja-Karlander E. Evaluation of orthodontic treatment after 1 year of retention—a randomized controlled trial. Eur J Orthod. 2010;32:542–7.

Edwards JG. A long-term prospective evaluation of the circumferential supracrestal fiberotomy in alleviating orthodontic relapse. Am J Orthod Dentofac Orthop. 1988;93:380–7.

Gill DS, Naini FB, Jones A, Tredwin CJ. Part-time versus full-time retainer wear following fixed appliance therapy: a randomized prospective controlled trial. World J Orthod. 2007;8:300–6.

Hichens L, Rowland H, Williams A, Hollinghurst S, Ewings P, Clark S, Ireland A, Sandy J. Cost-effectiveness and patient satisfaction: Hawley and vacuum-formed retainers. Eur J Orthod. 2007;29:372–8.

Katsaros C, Livas C, Renkema AM. Unexpected complications of bonded mandibular lingual retainers. Am J Orthod Dentofac Orthop. 2007;132(6):838–41.

Levin L, Samorodnitzky-Naveh GR, Machtei EE. The association of orthodontic treatment and fixed retainers with gingival health. J Periodontol. 2008;79(11):2087–92.

Pandis N, Vlahopoulos K, Madianos P, Eliades T. Long-term periodontal status of patients with mandibular lingual fixed retention. Eur J Orthod. 2007;29(5):471–6.

Pratt MC, Kluemper GT, Hartsfield JK Jr, Fardo D, Nash DA. Evaluation of retention protocols among members of the American Association of Orthodontists in the United States. Am J Orthod Dentofac Orthop. 2011;140(4):520–6.

Rowland H, Hichens L, Williams A, Hills D, Killingback N, Ewings P, Clark S, Ireland AJ, Sandy JR. The effectiveness of Hawley and vacuum-formed retainers: a single-center randomized controlled trial. Am J Orthod Dentofac Orthop. 2007;132(6):730–7.

Sauget E, Covell DA, Boero RP, Lieber WS. Comparison of occlusal contacts with use of Hawley and clear overlay retainers. Angle Orthod. 1997;67(3):223–30.

Shawesh M, Bhatti B, Usmani T, Mandall N. Hawley retainers full- or part-time? A randomized clinical trial. Eur J Orthod. 2010;32(2):165–70.

Sinclair PM, Little RM. Maturation of untreated normal occlusions. Am J Orthod. 1983;83(2):114–23.

Singh P, Grammati S, Kirschen R. Orthodontic retention patterns in the United Kingdom. J Orthod. 2009;36(2):115–21.

Störmann I, Ehmer U. A prospective randomized study of different retainer types. J Orofac Orthop. 2002;63(1):42–50.

Sun J, Yu YC, Liu MY, Chen L, Li HW, Zhang L, Zhou Y, Ao D, Tao R, Lai WL. Survival time comparison between Hawley and clear overlay retainers: a randomized trial. J Dent Res. 2011;90(10):1197–201.

Tacken MP, Cosyn J, De Wilde P, Aerts J, Govaerts E, Vannet BV. Glass fibre reinforced versus multistranded bonded orthodontic retainers: a 2 year prospective multi-centre study. Eur J Orthod. 2010;32(2):117–23.

Taner T, Haydar B, Kavuklu I, Korkmaz A. Short-term effects of fiberotomy on relapse of anterior crowding. Am J Orthod Dentofac Orthop. 2000;118(6):617–23.

Thickett E, Power S. A randomized clinical trial of thermoplastic retainer wear. Eur J Orthod. 2010;32:1–5.

Valiathan M, Hughes E. Results of a survey-based study to identify common retention practices in the United States. Am J Orthod Dentofac Orthop. 2010;137(2):170–7.

Maintenance of Fixed Appliances During Treatment

12

The length of a course of orthodontic treatment is variable and chiefly contingent on the objectives, compliance and operator parameters. However, the average duration for fixed appliance-based treatment has been estimated at 20 months (Tsichlaki et al. 2016). During this period, it is essential that there is a commitment to maintaining optimal dental health and care of fixed appliances. Suboptimal appliance care and compliance may lead to extended duration of treatment and increase risk of common iatrogenic effects of orthodontics including enamel demineralisation and adverse periodontal effects.

Prior to commencing fixed appliance treatment, recording of baseline levels of oral hygiene, dietary habits and smoking history are helpful. A plaque score of no more than 20% is considered a prerequisite before instituting treatment. A basic periodontal examination (BPE) should also be undertaken, and where a Code 3 is recorded, a full 6-point pocket charting of the affected sextant is carried out supplemented with appropriate radiographic images such as periapicals. This information allows evaluation of the risk of developing both enamel demineralisation and loss of periodontal attachment. Importantly, it also allows the provision of appropriate advice, information and management at the beginning, during and following completion of treatment.

During the placement of fixed appliances, every attempt should be made to ensure that the risk of possible iatrogenic effects is limited. In particular, following manufacturers' material recommendations and bonding techniques to reduce the risk of debonding of attachments is important. Equally, opening the bite to limit or remove direct occlusal contacts on fixed appliance attachments, removal of residual composite around attachments that may otherwise promote plaque accumulation and ensuring archwire ends are cut flush to molar tubes or wire components tucked away from the soft tissues are all sensible approaches to reducing the risk of discomfort and breakages.

P. Fleming, J. Seehra, *Fixed Orthodontic Appliances*, BDJ Clinician's Guides,
https://doi.org/10.1007/978-3-030-12165-5_12

Mechanical plaque removal techniques are paramount around fixed appliances reducing the risk of developing both white spot lesions (Box 12.1) and periodontal inflammation (Box 12.2). Cleaning of teeth and appliance is recommended a minimum of twice daily and ideally after every meal using either a modified Bass or scrub technique when using manual toothbrushes. The efficacy of plaque removal with toothbrushing could be increased with the use of both disclosing tablets (Fig. 12.1a, b) and interdental brushes. Recently, the use of electric toothbrushes has increased in popularity; these do appear to be more effective in terms of plaque control than manual, although the clinical importance of this remains unclear (Yaacob et al. 2014). Although the evidence is inconclusive, electric brushes may be helpful in reducing gingivitis in patients undergoing orthodontic treatment (Kaklamanos and Kalfas 2008).

Clear instructions should be given in relation to avoidance of breakages of the appliance and methods to maintain optimal dental health given. At each adjustment visit, the level of oral hygiene and appliance care should be assessed and oral hygiene instructions reinforced with positive encouragement, as required. Routine dental appointments and where indicated attendance with a dental hygienist should be advocated throughout the course of orthodontic treatment.

The practical steps involved in maintaining optimal dental health and appliance care during fixed appliance treatment are outlined below.

Box 12.1 Demineralisation (White Spot Lesions)

Demineralisation (white spot lesions) occurs due to a loss of mineralised tooth substance and results from an interaction between tooth surfaces harbouring plaque deposits with specific acid-forming bacteria found within the oral cavity, dietary sugar intake and time. A broad range of incidence (2–96%) has been reported in the literature with at least one tooth affected in up to 50% of patients undergoing fixed appliance-based orthodontics (Gorelick et al. 1982) (Fig. 12.1c–e). In addition to dietary advice (Box 12.4), topical fluoride supplements can be utilised to mitigate against the development of lesions in orthodontic patients. In patients undergoing fixed appliance treatment, the daily use of 0.05% sodium fluoride mouthrinse (Colgate™) preferably alcohol-free is advocated (Benson et al. 2004) (Fig. 12.1f). Recently, casein phosphopeptide-amorphous calcium phosphate (CPP-ACP)-based products have been shown some promise in reducing white spot lesions during treatment (Robertson et al. 2011). The management protocols for white spot lesions following orthodontic treatment are lacking. Historically, slow remineralisation with saliva and maintenance of a high level of oral hygiene were recommended (Ogaard et al. 1988) (Fig. 12.2a–c). However, prospective investigations have suggested superior results with a monthly application of a fluoride varnish over a 6-month period (He et al. 2016). The benefit of CPP-ACP following orthodontics in promoting remineralisation seems to be equivocal (Huang et al. 2013).

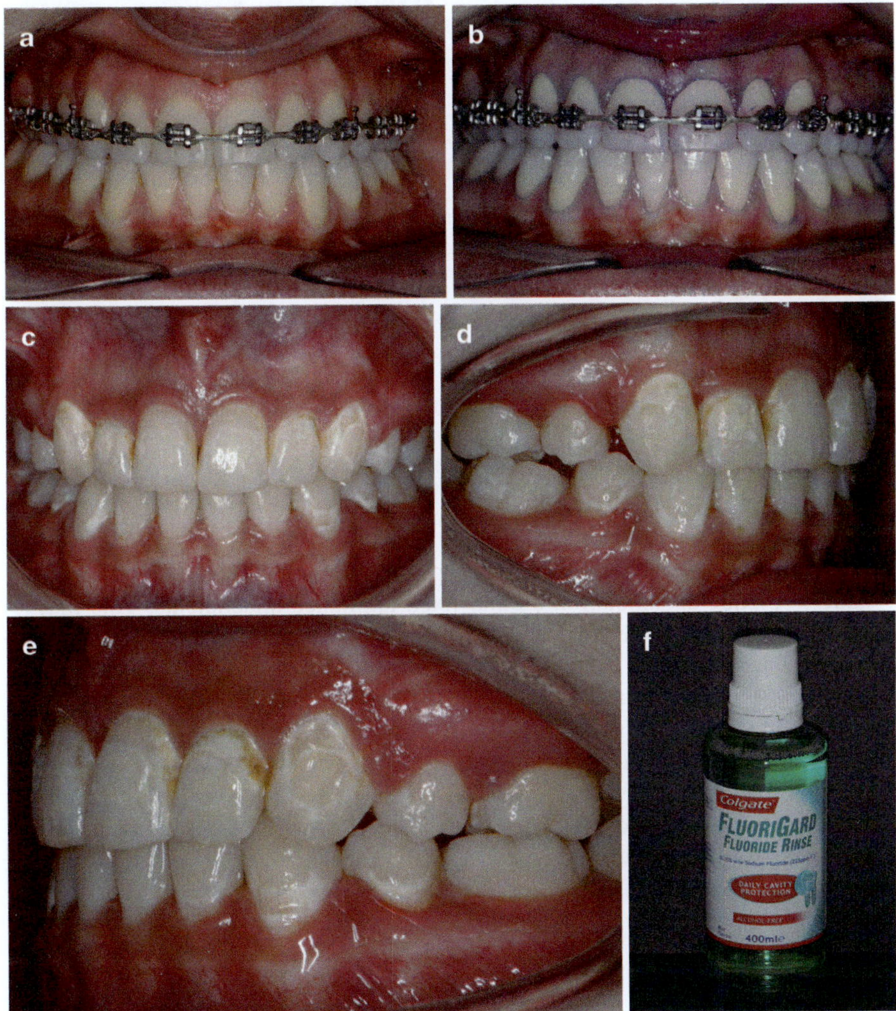

Fig. 12.1 (**a–f**) Plaque disclosure can be useful to highlight stagnation areas (**a**, **b**). Demineralisation during treatment leading to diffuse white and brown areas (**c–e**). Daily use of fluoride mouthrinse (0.05%) during active treatment can help to reduce the risk of demineralisation (**f**)

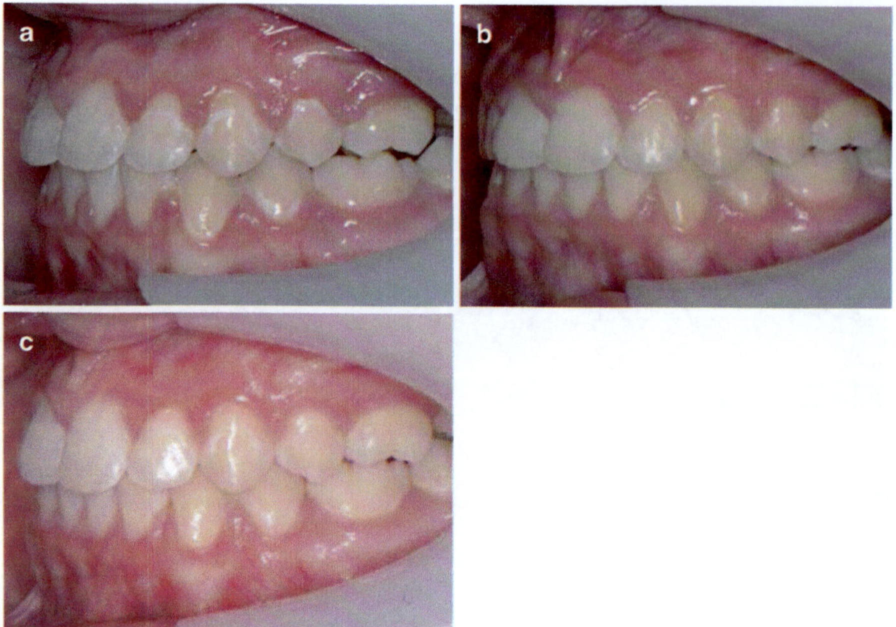

Fig. 12.2 (**a–c**) Demineralisation tends to improve with excellent oral hygiene following removal of appliances

Box 12.2 Gingival Inflammation

Gingival inflammation during fixed appliance treatment occurs commonly due to plaque accumulation around fixed appliance attachments. This may well be accompanied by demineralisation in view of the common causal pathway related to plaque control (Fig. 12.3a–c). Failure to control inflammation can lead to progression with irreversible changes including loss of alveolar bone and periodontal attachment (Bollen et al. 2008) in susceptible patients. Overall, the mean amount of attachment loss is considered to be negligible with 0.11 mm reported (Papageorgiou et al. 2018); however, it is important that treatment is not commenced until active disease is controlled and that preventative measures are in place.

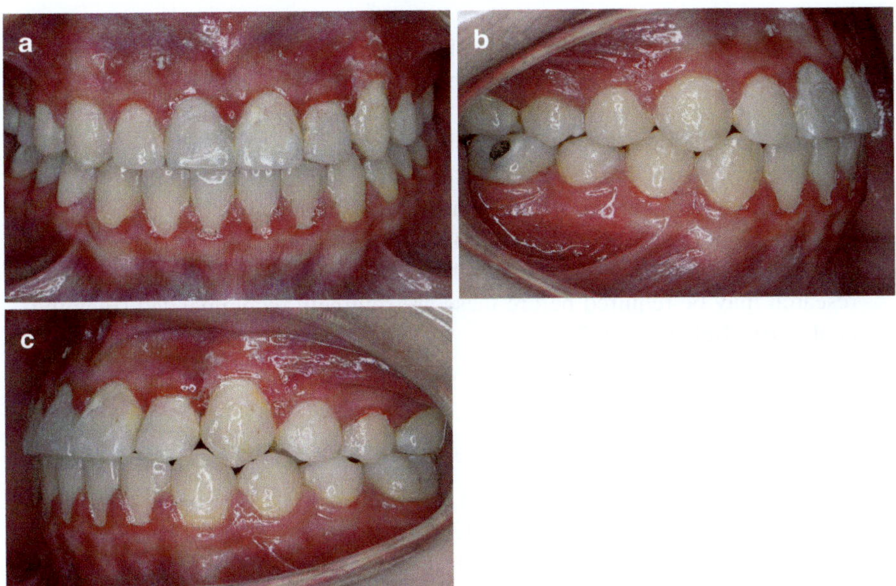

Fig. 12.3 (**a–c**) A combination of gingivitis and demineralisation following orthodontic debond

Box 12.3 Pain Control

Pain and discomfort are almost pervasive during orthodontics, typically peaking during the initial stages, either after separator placement or initial activation of a fixed appliance (Jones and Chan 1992). Overall, pain has been reported at some stage during treatment by 91% of patients and following each appointment by 39%, although its intensity may subside at later appliance adjustments (Johal et al. 2018). In terms of severity, pain subsequent to initial appliance placement is thought to be more sustained and severe than that attributed to dental extractions, with orthodontic pain typically lasting of the order of 4–5 days longer and being of higher intensity in most cases (Jones and Chan 1992). The prospect of pain is known to deter potential candidates for orthodontics (Trulsson et al. 2002). Furthermore, treatment discontinuation has been attributed to discomfort experienced in the early stages of appliance therapy (Patel 1992).

Orthodontic pain may be elicited by heavy pressure placed on the tooth by normal mastication, or it may arise spontaneously. It is known to be influenced by psychological, sociocultural and environmental factors, making objective evaluation difficult. Nonlinear relationships have been shown between pain after initial archwire placement and archwire material and age, social class, degree of force applied, dental arch relationships and dental crowding (Jones and Chan 1992). However, it is sensible to counsel patients that pain is highly likely, particularly for the first 7 days after appliance placement and after further manipulation, particularly following insertion of stiffer stainless steel wires (Johal et al. 2018) and to recommend pharmacological control, as required. Non-steroidal anti-inflammatories have proven marginally more effective than paracetamol for orthodontic pain and should therefore be recommended in suitable patients (Monk et al. 2017). A range of non-pharmacological agents, including lasers and masticatory aids (including chewing gum) have shown potential benefit in pain control, although further research may be required before these are routinely recommended (Fleming et al. 2016; Ireland et al. 2016).

Box 12.4 Dietary Advice

There is some evidence that diet can improve as a result of fixed appliance-based orthodontics (Johal et al. 2013). Dietary control is also important in order to reduce the risk of demineralisation and caries, as well as the likelihood of breakages. Multiple breakages during treatment may lengthen the duration of treatment (Skidmore et al. 2006) and increase the risk of iatrogenic damage to the dental tissues. Causes of appliance breakages include dietary components including particularly sticky and tough foodstuffs and habits such as nail-biting and pen-chewing. Softer foods which require less chewing can be encouraged particularly in the initial days after appliance placement. Typically, hard and sticky food such as pizza crust, toffees, biscuits, nuts and raw vegetables should be avoided or in some cases can be modified into smaller portions. Consumption of excessive carbonated drinks and fruit juices, particularly in conjunction with inadequate plaque control, will increase the risk of white spot lesions (Box 12.1).

12.1 Maintenance of Fixed Appliances During Treatment: Practical Steps

During the course of fixed appliance treatment, patients tend to become more resistant to soft tissue irritation from the appliance itself. However, when the appliance is first placed, soft tissue trauma from sharp components such as the end of lacebacks which have not been tucked towards the teeth (Fig. 12.4a), bracket hooks or excess archwire protruding from the end of the molar tubes is commonplace. To help with this transition, orthodontic relief wax (Fig. 12.4b–g) or silicone-based

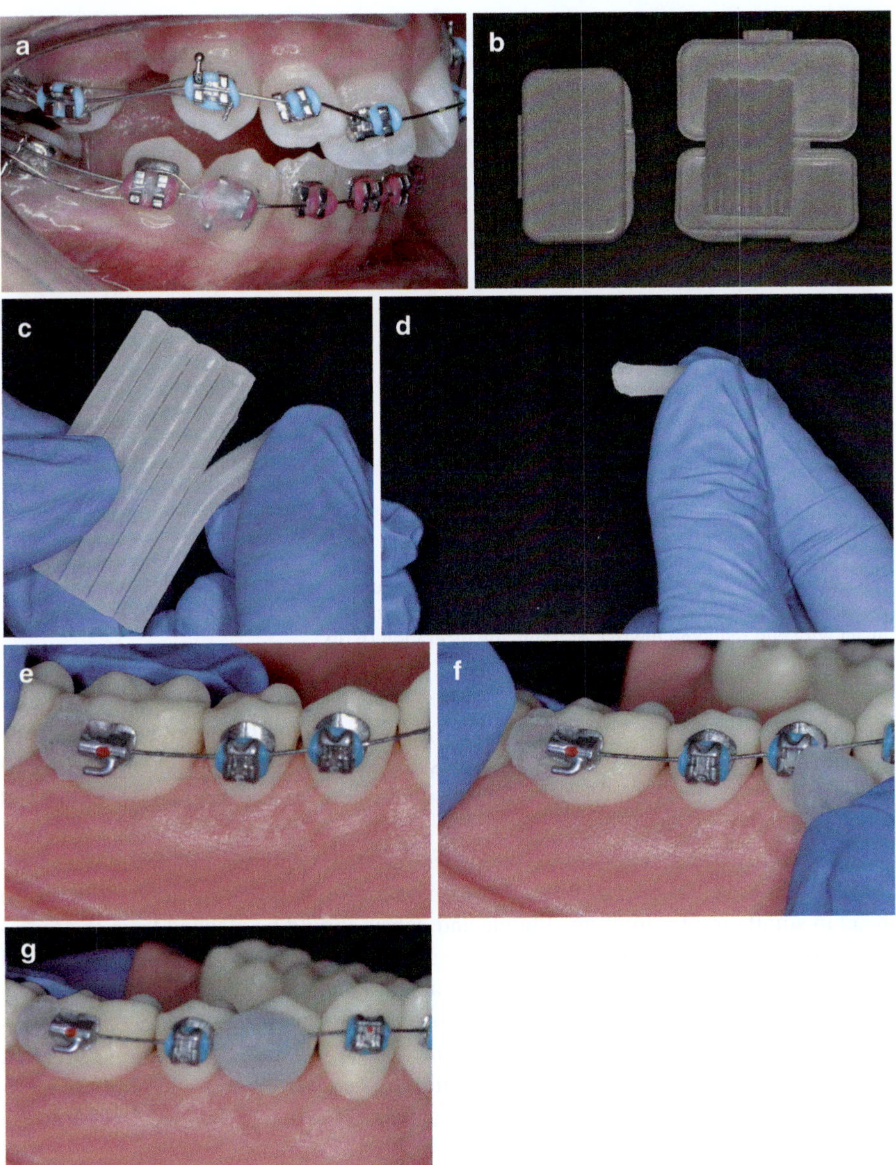

Fig. 12.4 (**a–g**) Use of relief wax to obscure sharp areas and enhance comfort, particularly during the early stages of treatment

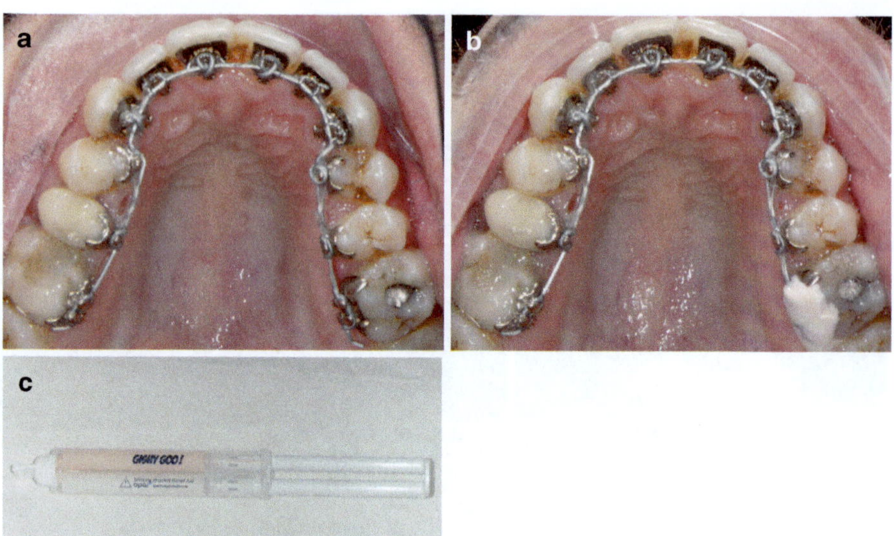

Fig. 12.5 (**a–b**) Upper Incognito™ appliance with wire overextended in UL6 region, while UR6 has been cinched adequately (**a**). Gishy Goo™ has been placed in the UL6 region to obscure the distal wire end reducing the risk of traumatic ulceration (**b**, **c**)

material (e.g. Gishy Goo ™; Fig. 12.5a–c) can be placed directly on the appliance to reduce any discomfort. It may be necessary to dry the area prior to placing the wax. Patients should be advised to remove the wax prior to eating and drinking and to replace intermittently.

The modified Bass technique can be recommended with the bristles of the toothbrush held at a 45-degree angle to the gingival margin while moving the toothbrush head in small circular motions. Plaque and debris should be cleaned from the gingival margins, buccal, lingual and occlusal surfaces of the teeth (Fig. 12.6a–f) as well as surrounding the appliance components and attachments. The latter is particularly important as demineralisation is known to occur surrounding the attachments particularly in less accessible areas including the lateral incisor-canine region (Gorelick et al. 1982). Both single-tuft and interdental brushes can be placed under the archwires to debride the margins around the brackets as these may be inaccessible to the larger head of a toothbrush (Fig. 12.6g–j).

Interproximal cleaning between the teeth can be facilitated by interdental brushes and dental floss. Interdental brushes are available in a range of different sizes (Fig. 12.7a). During treatment, the dimensions between contact points of teeth and access to these areas can change, and the appropriate brush size may need to change accordingly (Fig. 12.7b, c). In particularly tight contact point regions, dental 'super-floss' may be used to aid interproximal cleaning (Fig. 12.7d–h).

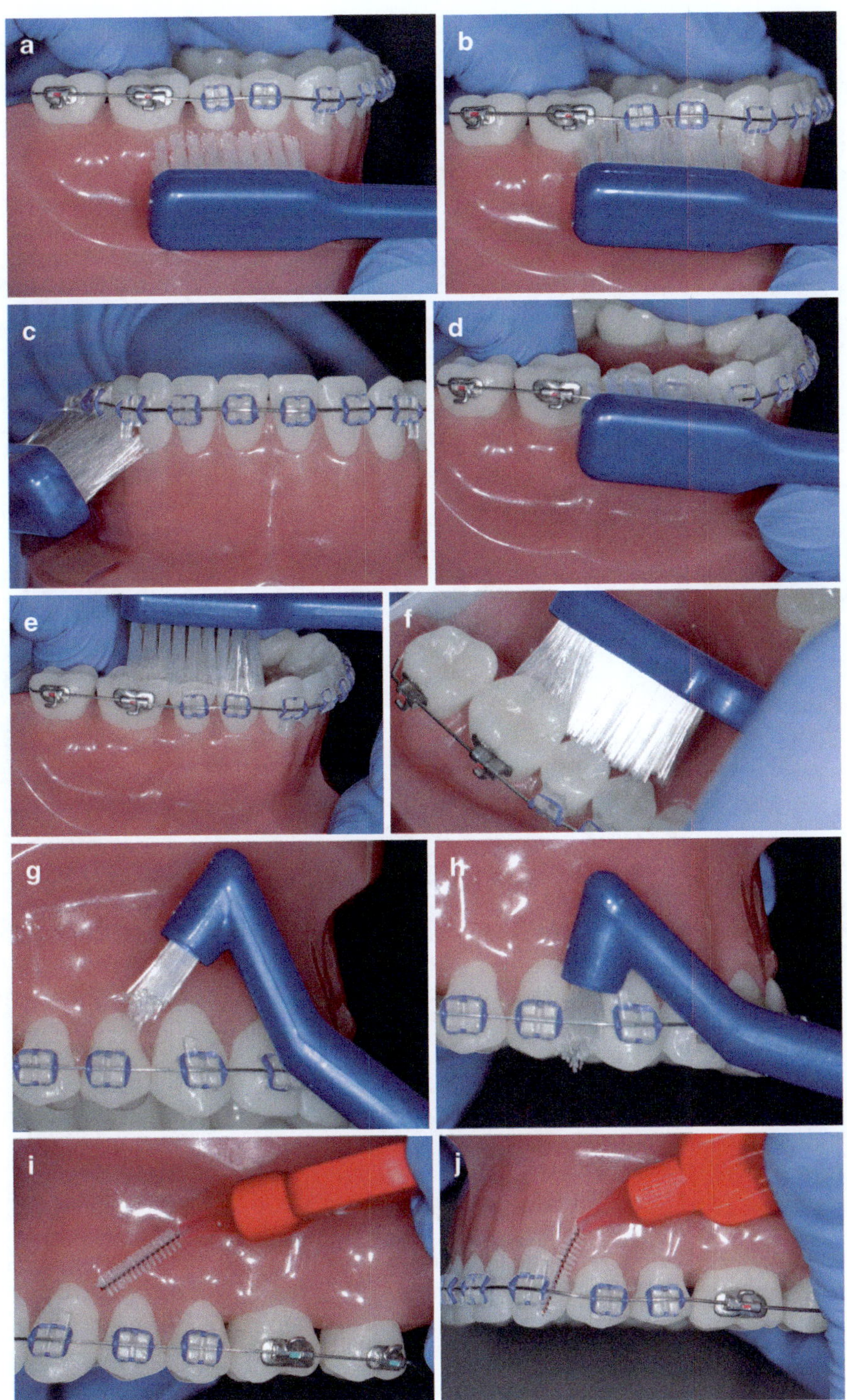

Fig. 12.6 (**a–j**) Oral hygiene measures to optimize plaque control particularly gingival to the attachments and beneath the arch wire

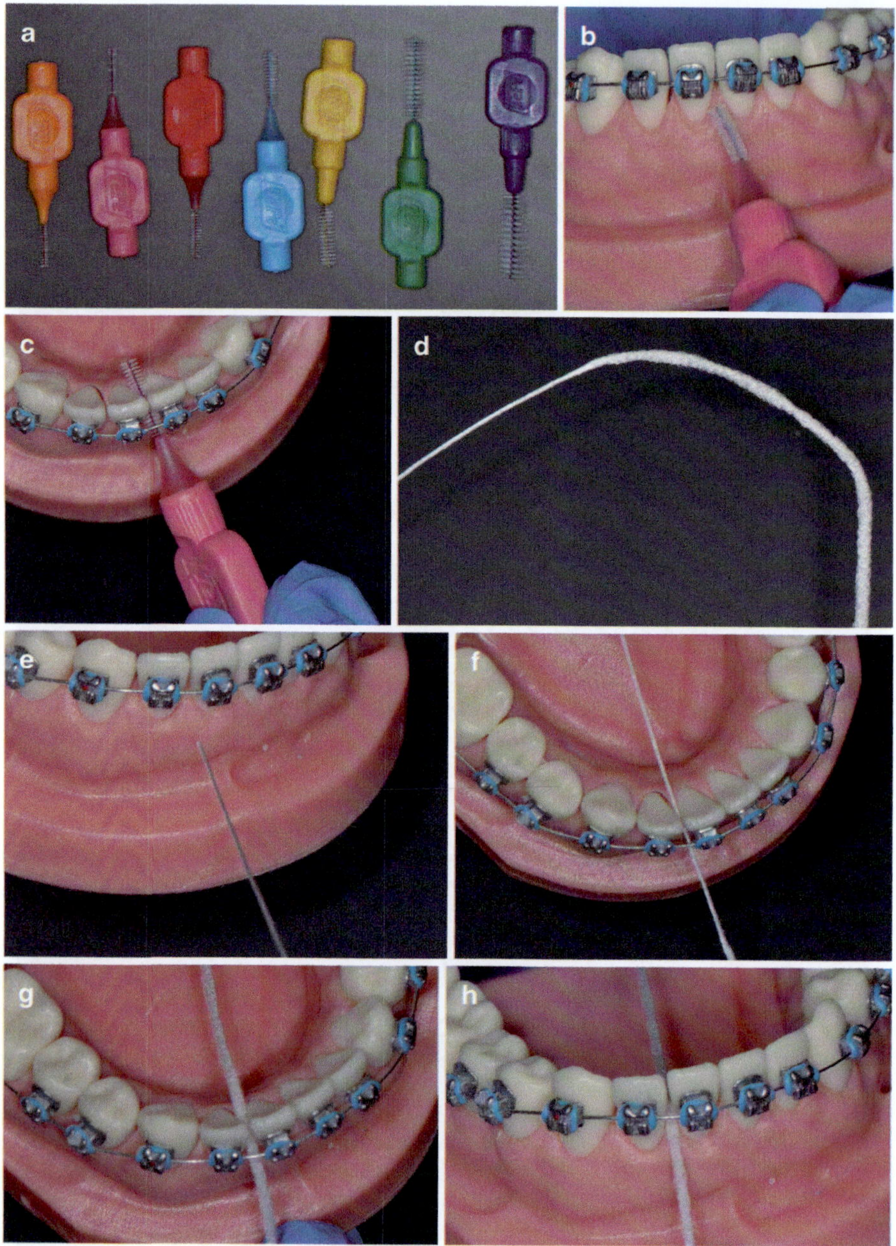

Fig. 12.7 (**a–h**) Use of inter-proximal brushes and SuperFloss™ to facilitate inter-proximal cleaning

References

Benson PE, Parkin N, Millett DT, Dyer FE, Vine S, Shah A. Fluorides for the prevention of white spots on teeth during fixed brace treatment. Cochrane Database Syst Rev. 2004;(3):CD003809. Review.

Bollen AM, Cunha-Cruz J, Bakko DW, Huang GJ, Hujoel PP. The effects of orthodontic therapy on periodontal health: a systematic review of controlled evidence. J Am Dent Assoc. 2008;139(4):413–22.

Fleming PS, Strydom H, Katsaros C, et al. Non-pharmacological interventions for alleviating pain during orthodontic treatment. Cochrane Database Syst Rev. 2016;12:CD010263.

Gorelick L, Geiger AM, Gwinnett AJ. Incidence of white spot formation after bonding and banding. Am J Orthod. 1982;81(2):93–8.

He T, Li X, Dong Y, Zhang N, et al. Comparative assessment of fluoride varnish and fluoride film for remineralization of postorthodontic white spot lesions in adolescents and adults over a 6-month period: a single-center, randomized controlled clinical trial. Am J Orthod Dentofac Orthop. 2016;149(6):810–9.

Huang GJ, Roloff-Chiang B, Mills BE, et al. Effectiveness of MI Paste Plus and PreviDent fluoride varnish for treatment of white spot lesions: a randomized controlled trial. Am J Orthod Dentofac Orthop. 2013;143(1):31–41.

Ireland AJ, Ellis P, Jordan A, et al. Comparative assessment of chewing gum and ibuprofen in the management of orthodontic pain with fixed appliances: a pragmatic multicenter randomized controlled trial. Am J Orthod Dentofac Orthop. 2016;150(2):220–7.

Johal A, Abed Al Jawad F, Marcenes W, Croft N. Does orthodontic treatment harm children's diets? J Dent. 2013;41(11):949–54.

Johal A, Ashari AB, Alamiri N, et al. Pain experience in adults undergoing treatment: a longitudinal evaluation. Angle Orthod. 2018;88(3):292–8.

Jones M, Chan C. The pain and discomfort experienced during orthodontic treatment: a randomized controlled clinical trial of two initial aligning arch wires. Am J Orthod Dentofac Orthop. 1992;102(4):373–81.

Kaklamanos EG, Kalfas S. Meta-analysis on the effectiveness of powered toothbrushes for orthodontic patients. Am J Orthod Dentofac Orthop. 2008;133(2):187.e1–14.

Monk AB, Harrison JE, Worthington HV, Teague A. Pharmacological interventions for pain relief during orthodontic treatment. Cochrane Database Syst Rev. 2017;11:CD003976. https://doi.org/10.1002/14651858.CD003976.pub2.

Ogaard B, Rølla G, Arends J, ten Cate JM. Orthodontic appliances and enamel demineralization. Part 2. Prevention and treatment of lesions. Am J Orthod Dentofac Orthop. 1988;94(2):123–8.

Papageorgiou SN, Papadelli AA, Eliades T. Effect of orthodontic treatment on periodontal clinical attachment: a systematic review and meta-analysis. Eur J Orthod. 2018;40(2):176–94.

Patel V. Non-completion of active orthodontic treatment. Br J Orthod. 1992;19(1):47–54.

Robertson MA, Kau CH, English JD, Lee RP, Powers J, Nguyen JT. MI Paste Plus to prevent demineralization in orthodontic patients: a prospective randomized controlled trial. Am J Orthod Dentofac Orthop. 2011;140(5):660–8.

Skidmore KJ, Brook KJ, Thomson WM, Harding WJ. Factors influencing treatment time in orthodontic patients. Am J Orthod Dentofac Orthop. 2006;129(2):230–8.

Trulsson U, Strandmark M, Mohlin B, Berggren U. A qualitative study of teenagers' decisions to undergo orthodontic treatment with fixed appliance. J Orthod. 2002;29(3):197–204.

Tsichlaki A, Chin SY, Pandis N, Fleming PS. How long does treatment with fixed orthodontic appliances last? A systematic review. Am J Orthod Dentofac Orthop. 2016;149(3):308–18.

Yaacob M, Worthington HV, Deacon SA, et al. Powered versus manual toothbrushing for oral health. Cochrane Database Syst Rev. 2014;(6):CD002281.

References

Index

P. Fleming, J. Seehra, *Fixed Orthodontic Appliances*, BDJ Clinician's Guides,
https://doi.org/10.1007/978-3-030-12165-5

The manufacturer's authorised representative in the EU is Springer Nature Customer Service Centre GmbH, Europaplatz 3, 69115 Heidelberg, Germany. If you have any concerns regarding our products, please contact ProductSafety@springernature.com

Printed and bound by CPI Group (UK) Ltd, Croydon, CR0 4YY
23/07/2026
02175589-0001